Recent Results in Cancer Research

Fortschritte der Krebsforschung

Progrès dans les recherches sur le cancer

37

Springer-Verlag New York · Heidelberg · Berlin 1971

Recent Results in Cancer Research

Fortschritte der Krebsforschung

Progrès dans les recherches sur le cancer

37

Edited by

V. G. Allfrey, New York · M. [illegible], Basel · K. [illegible]
A. [illegible], [illegible] · F. [illegible] · [illegible]
W. [illegible], [illegible] · N. N. [illegible] · [illegible]
P. [illegible], [illegible] · A. V. [illegible] · [illegible]
C. J. Cunningham, Richmond · [illegible] · [illegible]
G. Della Porta, Milano · P. [illegible] · [illegible]
H. [illegible], New York · [illegible] · [illegible]
R. J. C. Harris, Salisbury · [illegible] · [illegible]
[illegible], Lyon · W. C. [illegible] · [illegible]
[illegible], New York · [illegible] · G. Klein, Stockholm
H. Koprowski, Philadelphia · [illegible], New York · [illegible]
G. Mathé, Villejuif · [illegible] · [illegible]
V. R. Potter, Madison · [illegible] · [illegible]
E. A. Saxén, Helsinki · C. G. [illegible] · [illegible]
W. Szybalski, Madison · [illegible] · [illegible]
A. Tissières, Genève · [illegible] · [illegible]
T. [illegible]

Editor in chief

P. Rentchnick, Genève

Springer-Verlag New York · Heidelberg · Berlin 1971

S. Chiappa · R. Musumeci · C. Uslenghi

Endolymphatic Radiotherapy in Malignant Lymphomas

With Contributions by

G. Bonadonna · B. Damașcelli · G. Fava · F. Pizzetti · U. Veronesi

With 83 Figures

Springer-Verlag New York · Heidelberg · Berlin 1971

Sponsored by the Swiss League against Cancer

ISBN-13: 978-3-642-80604-9 e-ISBN-13: 978-3-642-80602-5
DOI: 10.1007/ 978-3-642-80602-5

Softcover reprint of the hardcover 1st edition 1971

 Typesetting, printing and binding: Konrad Triltsch, Graphischer Betrieb, 87 Würzburg, Germany.

Foreword

Clinical trials with Lipiodol ^{131}I were started in 1961 by my associate, S. CHIAPPA, and a group of physicians at the Institute of Radiology and the National Cancer Institute in Milan and development has been vigorously pursued during the past years. Once the rationale of this method was established, various aspects of the problem have been investigated, particularly the distribution of the radioactive dye into the lymph nodes as well as its fate and dosimetry in the body tissues. This monograph describes the extensive clinical evaluation and the radiological results obtained in a large group of patients with malignant lymphomas.

Endolymphatic radiotherapy as a therapeutic tool employing radionuclides has aroused interest at several meetings concerned with lymphology. In the recent monograph "Lymphography in cancer" by W. A. FUCHS, J. W. DAVIDSON and H. W. FISCHER, Dr. JANTET wrote a chapter on this specific subject. Many aspects are still debated, i. e. the choice of radionuclide, the specific clinical indications and the proper evaluation of the therapeutic effects.

It is hoped that further studies will come to more precise conclusions.

Whatever the future of endolymphatic radiotherapy in the field of clinical oncology, I want to call the attention of readers to the monograph of S. CHIAPPA and his coworkers. Their intelligent, exhaustive and critical work definitely constitutes, in my opinion, a useful contribution in this particular field. I wish also to acknowledge with thanks their remarkable contribution to the scientific activity of the Institute of Radiology.

Prof. ARDUINO RATTI, M. D.
Director, Istituto di Radiologia
University of Milan, Italy

Preface

In the fall of 1961, when I first injected a radioactive contrast material (Lipiodol Fluid ^{131}I) into the lymph vessels of the dorsum of the foot, it was in the belief that the isotope could be useful in following the distribution of the dye throughout the retroperitoneal lymph nodes, rather than for therapeutic purposes. The experience gained, first in animals and subsequently in man, suggested the possibility of using the radiation emission of ^{131}I for therapeutic purposes, too. It thus became possible for the first time to irradiate the lymphatic tissue and at the same time to check the results through periodical follow-up films.

Endolymphatic radiotherapy (ERT) has been used extensively in the past few years in several centers throughout the world. Both favorable results and criticism have helped to define its indications more precisely. After some nine years of experience with its use in the therapy of several types of neoplastic diseases, and especially of malignant lymphomas, I can state once more that endolymphatic radiotherapy is a therapeutic tool practically devoid of significant side effects. Since a good filling of the nodes is possible, particularly when the lymphatic tissue is not severely invaded by neoplastic cells, endolymphatic radiotherapy finds its principal indication as a prophylactic treatment for radiologically normal or suspicious lymph nodes below the diaphragm. In stage IV malignant lymphomas, however, where radiation therapy plays only a palliative role, endolymphatic radiotherapy can be used succesfully in combination with chemotherapy.

I believe that experiments and clinical trials with radioactive contrast materials of any kind could represent an interesting approach for treatment of cancer. I wish to thank all coauthors of this monograph, and in particular Dr. R. Musumeci and Dr. C. Uslenghi, whose diligence and competent work has contributed substantially in collecting the case material and in evaluating the results.

This book is dedicated to the memory of my father.

Sergio Chiappa

Acknowledgment

The authors wish to acknowledge with thanks the critical review of the manuscript by A. Ratti, M. D., Director of the Institute of Radiology, University of Milan, and P. Bucalossi, M. D., Director of the National Cancer Institute, Milan.

Contents

List of Authors

GIANNI BONADONNA, M. D., Clinical Associate, Clinical Chemotherapy Unit, National Cancer Institute, Milan

SERGIO CHIAPPA, M. D., Assistant Professor of Radiology, University of Milan; Chief, Radiological Department, Fatebenefratelli Hospital, Milan

BRUNO DAMASCELLI, M. D., Assistant Professor of Radiology, University of Milan

GIANNINO FAVA, Ph. D., Head, Section of Physics, National Cancer Institute, Milan

RENATO MUSUMECI, M. D., Assistant Professor of Radiology, University of Milan

FEDERICO PIZZETTI, M. D., Chief, Division of Pathology, National Cancer Institute, Milan

CARLO USLENGHI, M. D., Assistant Professor of Radiology, University of Milan; Clinical Assistant, National Cancer Institute, Milan

UMBERTO VERONESI, M. D., Head, Division of Clinical Oncology, National Cancer Institute, Milan

Chapter 1

Present Position of Radical and Palliative Treatment of Malignant Lymphomas

GIANNI BONADONNA

With 2 Figures

In the past decade advances in both diagnosis and treatment of malignant lymphomas, and particularly of Hodgkin's disease, have yielded a large amount of new information about their natural history, histopathologic classification and diagnostic evaluation, as well as new ideas concerning the basis for a rational therapeutic approach [46, 88, 100 a, 115, 123—125]. From a practical point of view, the most important result derived from all these studies is the fact that most physicians today, when facing the therapeutic problem, show greater optimism in their prognosis. Medical people are now aware that, contrary to what has for years been taught at universities and published, a malignant lymphoma need no longer be considered invariably fatal, but rather that adequate doses of radiation therapy in the early stages produce a high long-term survival rate, statistically compatible with cure [58, 63, 75, 91, 93, 99, 119].

The purpose of this introductory chapter is to outline briefly the modern concepts on radical and palliative therapy of malignant lymphomas. These new ideas are principally based on their histologic expression, mode of spread, meticulous diagnostic evaluation, both on admission and during the follow-up, and clinical classification.

1. Histopathologic Classification

For many years the histologic gradation of change proposed by JACKSON and PARKER in 1947, stressing the variation in malignant characteristics, has been widely accepted in differentiation between Hodgkin's paragranuloma, granuloma and sarcoma. Recently, the simplified LUKES classification [84, 85] has gained acceptance all over the world in view of the fact that preferential localizations and a distinct prognostic evolution vary according to the four fundamental histological expressions (Table 1.1). In fact, a retrospective clinical study according to histological type,

Table 1.1. *Terminology for the histologic expressions of Hodgkin's disease (proposed by the Nomenclature Committee, Rye, New York, September 13—15, 1966)* [106]

Histologic terms	Description
Lymphocytic predominance	A histocytic component of variable degree is usually found and represents a prominent component in approximately half of the cases. The process may be nodular or diffuse in histologic pattern. The group therefore includes not only the paragranuloma type of JACKSON and PARKER, where lymphocytes predominate, but also the lymphocytic and/or histocytic types, both nodular and diffuse of LUKES and BUTLER.
Nodular sclerosis	This histologic type is characterized by orderly bands of interconnecting collagenous connective tissue that subdivides distinctively abnormal lymphoid tissue, partially or entirely, into isolated cellular nodules.
Mixed cellularity	The histologic response in this group is intermediate between lymphocytic predominance and lymphocytic depletion and includes a complete variety of histologic components as follows: eosinophils, plasma cells, mature neutrophils, lymphocytes, hystiocytes and Reed-Sternberg cells, as well as variable not severe degrees of disorderly fibrosis without birefringent collagen formation.
Lymphocytic depletion	This group is composed of several histologic expressions of Hodgkin's disease that have in common lymphocytic depletion. It includes the diffuse fibrosis and reticular types of LUKES and BUTLER and the sarcoma type of JACKSON and PARKER.

made by KELLER et al. [72] on 176 cases, showed that the two largest groups were nodular sclerosis and mixed cellularity, while lymphocytic predominance and lymphocytic depletion occurred as much smaller entities. These results are very close to those published previously by HANSON [53], while in other series mixed cellularity appears to be the largest histologic group [34, 43]. Nodular sclerosis occurs mainly in patients with cervical and mediastinal involvement [29, 43, 53, 72]. Lymphocytic predominance occurs almost always in patients with stage I and II, while lymphocytic depletion and mixed cellularity in stages III and IV and are often associated with systemic symptoms [34, 72]. Lymphocytic predominance and nodular sclerosis have a favourable prognosis with prolonged median survival time in comparison to mixed cellularity and lymphocytic depletion [61 a, 72]. Finally, non-continuous dissemination occurs more often in the mixed cellularity and lymphocytic depletion types [72].

For lymphosarcoma and reticulum cell sarcoma, a less well defined histologic description is available at the present moment. Usually, lymphosarcoma is morphologically classified as lymphocytic and lymphoblastic, and reticulum cell sarcoma as differentiated or undifferentiated. Lymphoblastic lymphosarcoma and undifferentiated reticulum cell sarcoma are associated with a poorer prognosis. A particular type of lymphosarcoma is the giant follicle lymphosarcoma or Brill-Symmers' disease which in comparison to other types of malignant lymphomas has a fairly benign prognosis.

2. Clinical Classification

The importance of an internationally accepted clinical classification for malignant lymphomas was emphasized particularly at the Symposium on the Radiotherapy of Hodgkin's disease held in Paris in 1965 [123]. In fact, the variability of staging criteria appearing in the literature has been increasing in the past few years. A special Committee [106], whose members are competent clinicians in this field, proposed during another meeting held in Rye in 1965 a four-stage clinical classification

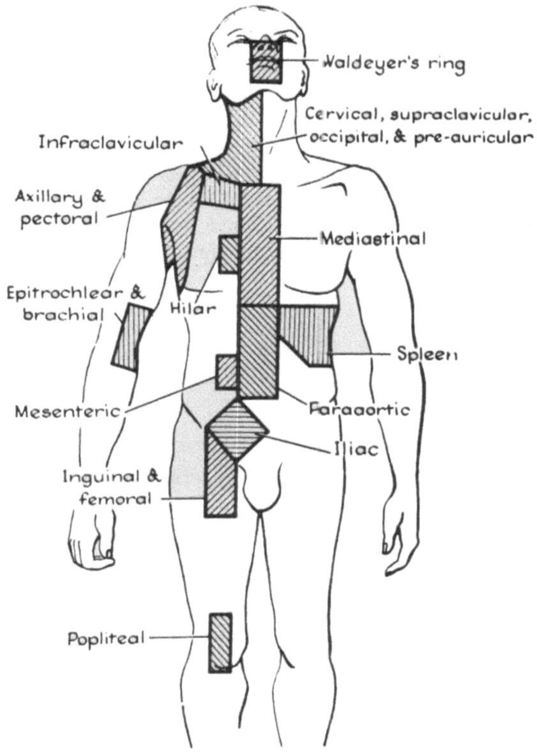

Fig. 1.1. Anatomical regions for the staging of Hodgkin's disease (proposed by the Committee on the Staging of Hodgkin's disease, Rye, New York, September 13—15, 1966). Modified by Kaplan and Rosenberg [63])

for Hodgkin's disease (Table 1.2) and defined the anatomical lymph node-bearing regions (Fig. 1.1). This classification seems to be more adequate than that proposed by Vera Peters [96] and widely used since 1950. The Rye classification has gained general acceptance since it allows the inclusion of a larger number of patients into the potentially curable category and clearly differentiates the cases in which the disease is still confined to the lymph nodes from those with extranodal involvement.

Table 1.2. *International staging classification for Hodgkin's disease (proposed by the Committee on the Staging of Hodgkin's disease, Rye, New York, September 13—15, 1965)* [106]

Stage [a]	Description
I	Disease limited to one anatomic region (Stage I_1) or to two contiguous anatomic regions (Stage I_2) on the same side of the diaphragm.
II	Disease in more than two anatomic regions or in two non contiguous regions on the same side of the diaphragm.
III	Disease on both sides of the diaphragm, but not extending beyond the involvement of lymph nodes, spleen, and/or Waldeyer's ring.
IV [b]	Involvement of the bone marrow, lung parenchyma, pleura, liver, bone, skin, kidneys, gastrointestinal tract, or any tissue or organ in addition to lymph nodes, spleen, or Waldeyer's ring.

[a] All stages will be subclassified as "A" or "B" to indicate the absence or presence, respectively, of systemic symptoms (fever, night sweats and generalized pruritus).

[b] Patients with involvement of viscera or tissue (e. g. stomach, bowel, bone or skin) with no evident disease in the lymph nodes or spleen should not been included in any of the groups described and they should be listed separately in clinical reports.

3. Diagnostic Evaluation

A meticulous diagnostic evaluation is essential for every patient in whom malignant lymphoma has been confirmed by biopsy. A careful documentation of the anatomical extent of the disease as well as of peculiar signs of its activity (e. g. systemic symptoms) is of fundamental importance in planning proper treatment. Table 1.3 outlines the studies considered desirable for accurate staging.

Among the recent diagnostic procedures employed in the diagnostic evaluation of malignant lymphomas, the invaluable role of lower limb lymphography has been stressed in innumerable publications and symposia [22, 123—125]. This simple procedure, evaluated by several investigators in almost every part of the world, has substantially contributed to the definition of the actual clinical stage of the disease, thus distinguishing patients suitable for radical therapy from those candidates for palliative treatment only. Therefore its use is recommended in all stages of the disease where patients with primary involvement of Waldeyer's ring are included [7]. A more extensive discussion of the diagnostic value of lymphography can be found further on in this monograph. The retroperitoneal adenopathies can also be detected by ultrasonic inspection [30], while mediastinoscopy [11] has been found useful in lymphomas with primary onset in the mediastinum. Recently, the value of diagnostic laparotomy with splenectomy, multiple liver and retroperitoneal node biopsies has been found by Glatstein et al. [47 a] and Lovenbraun et al. [82 a] "a valuable procedure for the more precise delineation of intra-abdominal sites of involvement of Hodgkin's disease prior to the initiation of extended field megavoltage radiation therapy with curative intent" [47 a]. The indications of laparotomy are valid also for lymphoreticular sarcomas [7].

Table 1.3. *Clinical and laboratory studies desirable for accurate staging in malignant lymphomas*

1. Careful clinical history with special attention to the presence of systemic symptoms.
2. Complete physical examination with thorough examination of Waldeyer's ring.
3. Postero-anterior and lateral chest film, with whole lung tomograms in presence of hilar adenopathies; lateral film of the pharynx with tomograms in presence of involvement of Waldeyer's ring.
4. Skeletal survey to include at least the base of skull, the thoraco-lumbar spine and the pelvis.
5. Retroperitoneal studies to include lower extremity lymphography and, occasionally, an excretory urogram and a pneumoretroperitoneum with tomography.
6. X-ray of the gastrointestinal tract, especially in presence of a lymphoreticular sarcoma.
7. Peritoneoscopy with biopsy of liver and spleen in presence of abdominal masses, hepatomegaly and splenomegaly.
8. When ever possible, unless the disease is clearly diffuse to viscera and/or bone marrow, diagnostic laparotomy with splenectomy, liver and retroperitoneal node biopsies, is recommended.
9. Radioactive isotope scanning of liver and spleen in presence of hepatomegaly and splenomegaly.
10. Complete blood count including erythrocyte sedimentation rate. Bone marrow biopsy.
11. Liver function tests to include BSP and alkaline phosphatase.
12. Renal function tests to include a urinalysis and serum uric acid.
13. Documentation of cutaneous anergy.

4. Natural History and Mode of Spread

It is well known that malignant lymphomas can have their primary origin in practically every organ or tissue of the body. However, in Hodgkin's disease as well as in lymphosarcoma and in reticulum cell sarcoma (lymphoreticular sarcomas), painless cervical adenopathy is by far the most frequent initial presenting symptom [5, 6, 13, 14, 100, 107, 110]. The mediastinal and para-aortic space for Hodgkin's disease, and Waldeyer's ring for lymphoreticular sarcomas, respectively, are among the most important sites of primary involvement besides the cervical area (Table 1.4).

Some recent studies have shown that Hodgkin's disease and lymphoreticular sarcomas do not spread initially with the same pattern [5—7, 13, 14, 52, 98, 107,

Table 1.4. *Percentage of involvement of the different lymph node-bearing areas in untreated patients with primary involvement of lymph nodes and spleen evaluated by lymphography.* (From Banfi, Bonadonna, Carnevali, and Fossati-Bellani: Courtesy of Lymphology [6])

Nodal areas	Hodgkin's disease (99 patients) %	Lympho-reticular sarcomas (67 patients) %	Nodal areas	Hodgkin's disease (99 patients) %	Lympho-reticular sarcomas (67 patients) %
Cervical	41	27	Iliac	6	23
Axillary	10	16	Femoral	1	17
Mediastinal	20	6	Splenic	2	2
Para-aortic	20	9			

110]. In fact, there is evidence that an orderly progression in the spread occurs for the majority of patients with Hodgkin's disease through invasion of adjacent lymphoid regions [5, 6, 13, 14, 52, 107]. In case of noncontiguous involvement, the area most frequently skipped is the mediastinum. This type of study provides further evidence that Hodgkin's disease has a unicentric origin and in about 80% of cases spreads in a relatively predictable pattern to contiguous lymphatic areas (Table 1.5).

Table 1.5. *Percent of contiguous and non-contiguous involvement in untreated consecutive patients with Hodgkin's disease versus those with lymphoreticular sarcomas.* (From Banfi, Bonadonna, Carnevali, and Fossati-Bellani: Courtesy of Lymphology [6])

Histologic type		Involvement		Spread	
		No. of cases	Contiguous	No. of cases	Contiguous
Hodgkin's disease	without lymphography	73	54 (74%)	79	57 (72%)
	with lymphography	80	47 (59%)		
	Total	153	101 (66%)		
Lymphoreticular sarcomas	without lymphography	53	19 (36%)	44	20 (45%)
	with lymphography	54	18 (33%)		
	Total	107	37 (35%)		

The lymphographic studies emphasized that the disease may actually involve primarily the retroperitoneal nodes and then spread via the thoracic duct to the cervical regions [5, 38, 107]. For this reason, where there is primary involvement of the retroperitoneal space, vascular rather than lymphatic dissemination is obviously more likely to occur early. Besides the route thoracic duct—subclavian vein, vascular dissemination can occur in about 10% of patients (mostly with lymphocytic depletion) by direct invasion of the blood vessels at the level of the lymph nodes [19, 102].

Lymphoreticular sarcomas with primary lymph-node involvement seem to have a less predictable pattern of spread than Hodgkin's disease [5, 7, 13, 98]. In fact, in only about one third of patients does the disease tend to involve the contiguous lymphoid regions. Furthermore, after local radiation therapy the lymphoma spreads preferentially to extranodal sites. This could be due to early vascular invasion, although histopathologic studies are not yet available. Clinical and lymphographic studies [5, 7, 13] suggest that in a high percentage of cases these sarcomas may arise in lymphoid regions below the diaphragm (retroperitoneal nodes and gastrointestinal tract). Therefore, they could spread at an early stage through the thoracic duct to distant non-contiguous nodes and especially to the blood stream. This is especially likely in children [14, 105].

A recent comprehensive evaluation of lymphoreticular sarcomas, primarily in Waldeyer's ring [7] showed that this type of lymphoma has a high frequency rate both in comparison to other primary sites of the same disease and to other neoplasms of the same region. In the large series evaluated at the National Cancer Institute,

Milan, its overall incidence among primary sites was found to vary from 21% to 57%, reticulum cell sarcoma being about three times as frequent as lymphosarcoma [7]. The tonsils and the nasopharynx are often involved and the disease has a high tendency to spread initially to the contiguous cervical nodes. With the advent of lymphography it was found that about 30% of patients with disease apparently localized in Waldeyer's ring and in the neck nodes had abnormal retroperitoneal

Table 1.6. *Distribution according to the Rye classification of 225 cases of lymphoreticular sarcomas with primary involvement of Waldeyer's ring, showing the importance of lymphography.* (From BANFI, BONADONNA, CARNEVALI, MOLINARI, MONFARDINI, and SALVINI: Courtesy of Cancer [7])

Stage	Cases without lymphography		Cases with lymphography	
	No.	%	No.	%
I_1	30	19.9	7	9.5
I_2	91	60.3	22	29.7
II	8	5.3	10	13.5
III	9	5.9	24	32.4
IV	13	8.6	11	14.9
Total	151	100	74	100

adenopathies (Table 1.6). Furthermore, in 20% of patients involvement of the stomach was found either at the time of initial examination or within two years of the beginning of treatment. Although a larger amount of case material, adequately evaluated, is required to confirm these data, the hypothesis is that in these patients lymphoreticular sarcomas may arise at the same time in Waldeyer's ring and in the gastrointestinal tract and spread initially to the cervical and retroperitoneal nodes, respectively [7]. Relapses after local treatment practically always occurred within two years and largely in extranodal sites.

5. Therapeutic Approach

a) Surgery

Surgery has been advocated in the past for unifocal adenopathies in the cervical, axillary and inguinal regions [120]. A relatively small number of cases underwent radical dissection, but the results reported were satisfactory, the 5-year survival rate being in the range of 75—80% [25, 47, 94, 114]. At the present time, with high-energy radiation equipment available, the surgical treatment of stage I_1 has been practically abandoned because intensive irradiation of the upper or lower trunk lymphoid regions can yield equivalent results, and has the advantage of allowing a precautionary irradiation of the adjacent areas.

Surgery is indicated for primary lymphomas in the gastrointestinal tract [37, 81, 92] and in the lung [95]. The stomach is more often involved (61%) than the small

(27%) and large intestine (11.5%) and lymphosarcoma usually has a higher incidence than reticulum cell sarcoma, Hodgkin's disease and giant-follicle lymphosarcoma [81, 192]. The prognosis is not directly related to the microscopic pattern or the site of origin but rather to the anatomical extent of the disease (presence or absence of regional adenopathies). The overall 5-year survival rate is in the range of 40 to 50% after surgical treatment [81, 92]. A higher percentage of survival can be achieved, provided the regional lymph nodes are not involved and a course of radiotherapy and/or chemotherapy follows the operation [92]. In the lung, on the contrary, primary lymphosarcoma (82.6%) has a higher incidence than reticulum cell sarcoma (17.4%). The 5-year survival rates after surgery or radiotherapy were 43.9 and 41.6%, respectively, in the case material studied by Papaioannou [97], while a combination of both treatments gave a slightly better survival rate (46.2%).

Finally, surgery may be useful in other clinical situations, such as spinal cord compression. Preliminary laminectomy followed by radiotherapy is indicated when the onset of clinical manifestations is very rapid, with bowel and bladder incontinence, and in this case about 60% of patients derive significant neurological improvement from this sequence [130]. If, on the contrary, early diagnosis of epidural involvement is made (back or radicular pain, paresthesias, herpes zoster at the same level), the combination of preliminary intravenous HN2 (0.4 mg/kg) or vinblastine (0.20 mg/kg) followed a few hours later by a course of local radiotherapy (2000 to 3000 rads) including within the field four spinal segments above and below the level of compression, represents the treatment of choice. In fact, in cases of suspicious spinal cord compression, if a myelography is carried out promptly and this procedure is followed by HN2 and radiotherapy, neurological improvement can be achieved in about 90% of patients [130]. Surgery may occasionally be indicated to remove the spleen in some cases with secondary hypersplenism, or when there is evidence that this organ is the main site of sequestration and destruction of erythrocytes. The results of therapeutic splenectomy are controversial [94].

b) Radiation Therapy

For many years, and practically until 1950, the widespread opinion among clinicians, hematologists and radiotherapists was that virtually all malignant lymphomas, regardless of their morphologic expression, clinical stage and type of treatment, sooner or later had an invariably fatal outcome. In 1950 a major landmark was represented by Vera Peters' paper, "A study of survivals of Hodgkin's disease treated radiologically" [96]. The author, who is one of the most competent radiotherapists in this field, reported the first detailed series of patients surviving for 10 years after radiation therapy. Furthermore, she was able to demonstrate that intensive irradiation of the involved lymph nodes, combined with precautionary or prophylactic treatment of the apparently uninvolved lymphoid regions, could improve 5-year survival rates by about 15—20%.

Peters confirmed her results a few years later [97] on a larger group of cases (Table 1.7). The somewhat unexpected favourable long-term results achieved with adequate radiation therapy have in the past five years stimulated a number of centres to treat patients with localized malignant lymphomas more carefully and aggressively.

Table 1.7. *Long-term survival rates in Hodgkin's disease treated with radiation therapy from the four largest series presently available*

Author	Extent of disease	Survival rate (%)			
		5 years	10 years	15 years	20 years
PETERS [97]	Stage I	73	52	42	35
	Stage II A	90	67	43	39
	Stage II B	23	13	3	0
	Stage III	11	5	6	4
MUSSHOFF [91]	Stage I	75	45		
	Stage II	80	40		
	Stage III	42	25		
EASSON [36]	localized	53.5	44.1	38.9	
	generalized	19.6	13.4	12.6	
KAPLAN [63]	Stage I and II	83	83		

Table 1.8. *Long-term survival rates in lymphoreticular sarcomas treated with radiation therapy from the two largest series presently available*

Author	Extent of disease	Survival rate (%)		
		5 years	10 years	15 years
PETERS [97]	Stage I	51	43	36
	Stage II	23	14	11
	Stage III	5	0.7	0
EASSON [36]	Localized	51.6	48.9	48.9
	Generalized	12.9	7.9	7.9

This more optimistic attitude toward prognosis in early stages (Stages I and II) of Hodgkin's disease was further enhanced by the results published by E. EASSON [36, 63] and H. S. KAPLAN [63, 64]. EASSON, with X-ray treatment carried out with 250 kV machines, achieved similar survival rates in both Hodgkin's disease and lymphoreticular sarcoma with localized (Stage I and II) adenopathies. The better results achieved in Hodgkin's disease by PETERS, who used similar 250 kV equipment, are undoubtedly due to the supplemental irradiation of contiguous lymphatic areas clinically free of disease. The survival rate for lymphoreticular sarcomas in PETERS' and EASSON's series is, however, about the same (Table 1.8). This confirms what has been stressed before, i. e. the usual mode of spread in Hodgkin's disease is to adjacent lymph node groups, while this occurs in the minority of patients with lymphoreticular sarcomas primary in the lymph nodes. Therefore, precautionary irradiation of the adjacent lymphoid regions can substantially increase the survival rate only in Hodgkin's disease [99, 108]. KAPLAN's figures represent a step further in the radical and precautionary therapy of localized Hodgkin's disease. He introduced the concept of "mantle" field which permits entire chains of lymph nodes to be treated in continuity with the delivery of 4.000 rads in 4 weeks. The availability of megavoltage X-ray and gamma-ray beams from linear accelerators, betatrons and cobalt-60 teletherapy units has allowed this technological improvement. This new method of intensive and extended radiotherapy accounts for the higher 10-year survival rate obtained by KAPLAN in his first series of patients in comparison to the results obtained by PETERS and EASSON. It should be noted at this point that KAPLAN's patients were evaluated also with lymphography, so they were really Stage I and II, while in PETERS' and EASSON's series a certain number of cases undoubtedly had silent adenopathies below the diaphragm. PETERS' results at 5 and 10 years after radiotherapy were better when the patients were in Stage II A rather than in Stage I. This means that fewer patients with Stage II A had adenopathies in the retroperitoneal space in comparison to those with Stage I, where the single cervical adenopathy could represent a distant extension of the disease, the onset of which was probably in the para-aortic region (Table 1.7).

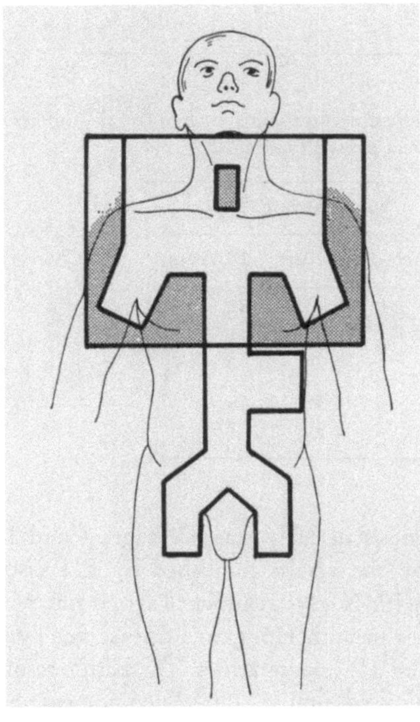

Fig. 1.2. Sketch of the radiation fields for the upper and the lower mantle. Anterior view

In conclusion, the present policy for treatment of Hodgkin's disease, localized either above or below the diaphragm (Stage I and II), is represented by intensive irradiation of all lymph node-bearing areas involved in association with adjacent clinically uninvolved lymphoid regions through the upper or lower trunk mantles (Fig. 1.2), with tumor doses ranging from 3,500 to 4,500 rads in about 4 weeks. The physical problem concerning the mantle fields has been discussed in several papers [48, 55, 113]. The clinical complications have usually been of minor importance, thus showing that megavoltage intensive treatment through such fields is tolerated very well. During treatment lungs, larynx, spinal cord and mandible are shielded. Skin reaction is negligible and esophagitis is transient. Bone marrow depression occurs, mainly during the lower trunk mantle irradiation, but reverts to normal within a few weeks in most cases. Occasionally, pericardial effusion has been observed [21, 27, 62]. This rationally planned intensive radiotherapy for clinically localized Hodgkin's disease offers a substantial chance of permanent cure to about 80% of patients, provided no systemic symptoms are present. As a definition of cure, that proposed by EASSON and RUSSEL can be adopted: "We can speak of cure when in time, probably a decade or so after treatment, there remains a group of disease-free survivors whose progressive death rate from all causes is similar to that of a normal population of the same sex and age constitution" [63]. KAPLAN observed recently that, after a mantle irradiation, if there is no recurrence within two years of initial treatment, it is practically not likely to occur during the following years [68]. This observation also fits in with our experience, i. e. if a patient is well and free of disease 2—3 years after initial irradiation, the possibility of a permanent cure is really very good.

When truly localized, the lymphoreticular sarcomas, if properly treated, can have a similar long-term survival rate as Hodgkin's disease [36, 128]. Since they tend to spread to adjacent lymphoid regions to a lesser extent than Hodgkin's disease, precautionary radiotherapy is not usually given. The regions involved are irradiated using megavoltage apparatus to the optimal tumor dose (3,500—4,500 rads) in approximately 4 weeks. Lymphoreticular sarcomas primary in Waldeyer's ring should receive a radical irradiation encompassing the whole of Waldeyer's ring and both cervical regions, even if the cervical nodes are not clearly palpable [7, 24]. In the large series of CARNEVALI and SALVINI [24], the survival rate was 38.9, 32.5 and 23.3% after 3, 5 and 10 years respectively from initial treatment, with a median survival of 18 months [23].

This analysis showed that the presence of cervical adenopathies considerably lowers the survival rate. In fact, while at 3, 5 and 10 years 65, 55 and 38% of patients were alive, these figures in the presence of affected cervical nodes were respectively 33, 29 and 20%.

Considering the tissue-dose administered, CARNEVALI and SALVINI observed a clear difference in survival time between the groups of patients adequately and inadequately treated (42% and 18% surviving respectively at 5 years). Finally, these authors did not find significant differences in terms of overall survival between lymphoreticular sarcomas with primary onset in Waldeyer's ring and in the lymph nodes. This group of patients, however, was not evaluated with lymphography.

Since the literature convincingly substantiates the argument that clinically localized malignant lymphomas are potentially curable in a very high percentage of cases after intensive irradiation, many centers throughout the world are at present employing a treatment plan, originally designed by KAPLAN [65, 67], with extended-field radical radiotherapy above and below the diaphragm in the attempt to achieve long-term results in stage III patients as well. Experience has already shown that this intensive and aggressive irradiation is tolerated impressively well [59, 60, 61, 65, 67]. Temporary leukopenia and thrombocytopenia occur in most cases, but the bone marrow function recovers within a rather short period of time [129], permitting the effective use of chemotherapy in the majority of patients who have relapsed with radiotherapeutically uncontrolled disease [61]. Since it is practically impossible to irradiate both upper and lower trunk mantles at the same time, the predominant site of disease should be the deciding factor. Ordinarily, treatment is initiated over the most heavily involved region, and treatment in this region is carried to completion before irradiation is started in other lymphoid regions (sequential technique). If the choice is not clear, it is wise to carry out first the irradiation in the lymphatics of the lower trunk, since a progression below the diaphragm can be a serious problem, and this region can be observed less easily than adenopathies above the diaphragm. In some instances with extensive involvement of both upper and lower lymphatics, as proposed by Kaplan [65], treatment to one trunk is interrupted after approximately 1500 rads; then the second trunk is irradiated also to about 1500 rads, following which treatment is carried to completion in the initial field and then in the other fields (alternating technique). As will be discussed in other chapters of this monograph, at the National Cancer Institute, Milan, we usually carried out the irradiation of the upper trunk lymphatics first, since the retroperitoneal adenopathies are opacified with Lipiodol I^{131}; after completion of the upper mantle, external irradiation was given to all lymphatic chains below the diaphragm.

Five or more years will probably be necessary to prove with certainty that the use of radiotherapy alone can either cure or markedly improve survival in a considerable percentage of patients with stage III lymphoma. From our experience and from what has been already published in the literature, it appears that extended-field radical radiotherapy can control Hodgkin's disease in an appreciable number of patients, provided there are no systemic symptoms. In patients with stage III B, the short-term results are less encouraging [67] and probably a course of chemotherapy should precede the course of radiotherapy. This sequence is the one we use at the National Cancer Institute, Milan, and is the treatment plan we advise for stage III B Hodgkin's disease. In lymphoreticular sarcomas with nodal involvement above and below the diaphragm, radiation therapy through extended fields should be given only after an adequate course of chemotherapy, even in the absence of systemic symptoms. Results of the attempt to control stage III lymphoreticular sarcoma with radiotherapy alone have been very poor in our experience. Therefore, the sequence chemotherapy—radiotherapy seems more advisable, since in the great majority of cases the disease has a tendency to spread to extranodal sites within a short period of time [5, 7, 13, 14].

In patients (Hodgkin's disease and lymphoreticular sarcomas) with stage IV radiation therapy plays a palliative role, and chemotherapy represents the treatment of choice. However, the contribution of radiotherapy should not be neglected, even where the disease is widespread, especially if bulky nodal masses or painful bone lesions are present. In some selected cases with e. g. initial invasion of the lung or of the skeleton, a fairly aggressive palliation is worthwhile.

c) Chemotherapy

Right from the time when chemotherapy was adopted for clinical purposes in medicine, immediately after World War II, it has proved very effective in controlling malignant lymphomas. Through many series of pharmacological and clinical studies the efficaciousness and the toxicity of the different drugs has been ascertained. At the present time, four classes of growth-inhibiting compounds are considered active and are therefore recommended for the treatment of lymphomas at an advanced stage: polyfunctional alkylating agents (including procarbazine) [20, 56, 73, 74, 86, 109, 126], vinca alkaloids [10, 12, 28, 39, 41, 57, 116, 131], antibiotics [15, 17, 18, 89, 104], and corticosteroids [51]. Table 1.9 shows the percentage of consistent objective responses and the average duration of regression that can be expected when the various agents are administered individually, respectively in Hodgkin's disease and in lymphoreticulosarcomas.

Table 1.9. *Percent response and mean duration which can be expected after adequate doses of different growth-inhibiting compounds in malignant lymphomas*

Drugs	Hodgkin's disease		Lymphoreticular sarcomas	
	Regression (%)	Mean duration (months)	Regression (%)	Mean duration (months)
Alkylating agents	80—90	6—12	60—70	4—12
Vinca alcaloids	60—65	5— 8	50—60	5— 6
Procarbazine	45—50	5— 6	30—35	4— 5
Antibiotics	45—55	2— 4	45—55	2— 4
Corticosteroids	40—60	2— 3	50—60	2— 2

Although it is recognized that chemotherapeutic treatment is suitable for every type of lymphoma at the fourth stage and, in association with radiologic treatment, in Hodgkin's disease at stage III B and in lymphoreticular sarcoma at stage III A and III B, various forms of treatment have been proposed in the last ten years.

For many years all authors agreed that the judicious use of all the effective drugs available, if adequately administered with a proper sequential schedule, by producing several consistent tumor regressions, could keep most patients active, relatively asymptomatic and in good general condition for long periods of time [16, 40, 45, 69, 121]. In more recent years, however, considerable efforts have been made to increase the frequency, magnitude and duration of regressions in malignant lymphomas by giving several drugs in combination.

In the sequential therapy scheme, patients receive a first therapeutic cycle with HN2 (0.4 mg/kg iv) or Thiotepa (0.8 mg/kg iv) or cyclophosphamide (4—6 gm/kg/course iv). Remissions can be continued for longer periods of time by maintenance of oral chemotherapy (chlorambucil 0.1—0.2 mg/kg/day and cyclophosphamide 100 to 200 mg/day), HN2, Thiotepa and chlorambucil seem more active in Hodgkin's disease, while cyclophosphamide has been reported to be more effective in lymphoreticular sarcomas. If and when the disease becomes refractory to the alkylating agents, one of the vinca alkaloids (vinblastine 0.10—0.15 mg/kg/week i.v. in Hodgkin's disease and vincristine 0.03—0.05 mg/kg/week i.v. in lymphoreticular sarcomas) is tried next, and then procarbazine (200—400 mg/day by mouth) if symptoms persist or recur. Recently, three antibiotics have been found useful in widespread malignant lymphomas. The methyl ester of streptonigrin (0.004 mg/kg/day for 6—8 weeks by mouth) has been reported to be useful in Hodgkin's disease [104] and equally effective as chlorambucil [7]. Daunomycin, adriamycin and bleomycin can produce a prompt response in both Hodgkin's disease and lymphoreticular sarcomas, although regressions are seldom complete and usually short-lived [15, 17, 18, 18 a, 25 a, 89]. Another alkylating agent 1,3-bis(chloroethyl) 1-nitrosourea (BCNU) has recently been found to be effective in about 50% of patients with Hodgkin's disease no longer responding to other anticancer agents [79, 103]. In pretreated patients. Methotrexate and actinomycin D alone are occasionally effective [50] while L-asparaginase seems useful only in some patients with lymphosarcoma [89].

A number of studies report the results of combination chemotherapy in Hodgkin's disease. Lacher and Durant [76] treated 16 patients with vinblastine plus chlorambucil and, although remissions occurred in 13 cases (81%), their mean duration was 7.5 months. DeVita and Serpick [32] treated 30 patients with a quadruple combination (vincristine, HN2, procarbazine and prednisone): 27 cases (90%) improved, but for a median duration of only 6 months. The same drug combination was administered by Bernard et al. [9] to a group of 67 patients with an 87% regression rate and an average duration of 2—19 months. A similar quadruple chemotherapy has been designed by Mathé et al. [4] with corticosteroids, vinblastine, TEM and procarbazine. Although an 86.2% remission rate was achieved at the expense of severe leukopenia, relapses occurred within a short period of time (of the 15 patients who had a complete remission, 8 relapsed within 4.2 weeks and 4 within 14 weeks). The quadruple combination proposed by Frei et al. [44, 90] employs cyclophosphamide, vincristine, Methotrexate and prednisone. Chemotherapy was given to 14 patients (7 with Stage I or II and 7 with Stage III). Patients with localized disease were also treated with radiation therapy and all but one entered a complete remission, not maintained for more than 30 months. Of the 7 patients with Stage III, 2 showed an induction failure, 2 died after 2 and 12 months respectively and 3 had a complete, non-maintained remission for 32, 33 and 35 months (2 patients also received X-ray treatment above the diaphragm).

The present data indicate that combination chemotherapy induces in patients with generalized Hodgkin's disease, especially if not previously treated, a high degree of complete remissions (80—90%). A similar response rate in untreated patients can also be achieved with HN2 alone [111], but a lesser number of cases shows the complete disappearance of all adenopathies. The real advantage of concurrent vs. sequential drug combination should be, besides the frequency of regressions, the magnitude and the duration of unmaintained remissions. The median duration of remissions after HN2 and maintenance therapy with chlorambucil was 8 months in Scott's series [111], while the total response rate to the sequence of vinblastine-cyclophosphamide or cyclophosphamide-vinblastine was approximately 80% with a median duration of maintained remission close to 10 months [23]. The trials with combination chemotherapy, as estimated from the published case material, with the exception of few patients with Stage III disease treated by Frei et al. [44, 99], do not yet prove that the duration of unmaintained remissions obtained with this method of treatment is greater than that achieved with single agents given in sequence and with maintenance therapy. Furthermore, the high regression rate obtained by Frei et al. in the 7 patients with localized Hodgkin's disease treated with radiotherapy and quadruple chemotherapy can be presently achieved with radical and prophylactic irradiation alone, without the addition of chemotherapy. This association does not seem from previous experiences to have a useful adjunctive role in increasing survival time [26, 70, 187] in localized cases without systemic symptoms.

Although all these published results do not provide sufficient evidence that combination chemotherapy is definitely superior to single sequential chemotherapy [16, 40], the more recent data of DeVita [33] and Serpick [112] emphasize that the percentage of long-term unmaintained complete remissions is really very high. In Hodgkin's disease [33] 43 patients have been treated since 1964 with HN2, vincristine, procarbazine and prednisone with an 81% complete remission (35 out of 43) and a median duration, calculated from the end of all therapies, of 18 months. Fifteen out of the 35 patients who had a complete remission relapsed with a median time to relapse of 11 months. The survival of the induction failures was 19 months and, for those 35 who entered a complete remission, 29 months. In lymphoreticular sarcomas [112] the same quadruple combination has been employed. In lymphosarcoma 7/15 patients entered into a complete remission with a median non-maintained duration of 13 months, while 3/8 reticulum cell sarcomas had a complete regression of 32 months. From these series there is a substantial evidence that the combination of effective agents increases the number of complete responses and prolongs the disease-free interval from the end of therapy. Other similar studies have been recently published [42, 54, 83, 92 a].

In conclusion, the question whether in advanced malignant lymphomas it is better to use chemotherapeutic agents in sequential or in concurrent combination still deserves more long-term study. At the present moment eradication of a malignant lymphoma can be achieved only by intensive irradiation, although prolonged remissions may be expected in an appreciable number of cases after intensive combination chemotherapy. (Tables 1.10 and 1.11) Nevertheless, a proper sequential rotation of useful drugs, can also allow the control of the disease for long periods of time in the majority of patients. Combination chemotherapy can be indicated in selected Stage II B—III B and IV patients, who should be preferably untreated and with a good

Table 1.10. *Schedule of drug administration (one cycle) adopted by the National Cancer Institute, Bethesda, USA. (33, 92 a, 112)*

Day	1	2	3	4	5	6	7	8	9	10	11	12	13	14	15—18
	HN2 6 mg/m² i. v.							HN2							
	VCR 1.4 mg/m² i. v.							VCR							No therapy
	Procarbazine 100 mg/m² p. o	—	—	—	—	—	—	—	—	—	—	—	—	→	
	Prednisone 40 mg/m² p. o.	—	—	—	—	—	—	—	—	—	—	—	—	→	

HN2: nitrogen mustard; VCR: Vincristine.

Patients: Hodgkin's disease and lymphoreticular sarcomas with advanced disease (generalized adenopathy and/or visceral involvement).

Treatment: Therapy consists of 6 2-weeks cycles with 2-week interval between each cycle. Therapy takes about 6 months to complete. Appropriate dosage attenuation schedule for bone marrow depression is indicated. The patients receive no maintenance therapy after the course of treatment.

Table 1.11. *Schedule of drug administration (one cycle) adopted by the National Cancer Institute, Milan, Italy (18 a)*

Day	1	2	3	4	5	6	7	8	9	10	11	12	13	14	15—28
	HN2 6 mg/m² i. v.													HN2	
	VCR 1.2 mg/m² i. v.													VCR	
	ADM 15 mg/m² i. v.	ADM	ADM												No therapy
							BLM 15 mg/m² i. v.	BLM	BLM	BLM					
	Prednisone 40 mg/m² i. m.	—	—	—	—	—	—	—	—	—	—	—	—	→	

HN2: nitrogen mustard; VCR: vincristine; ADM adriamycin; BLM: bleomycin.

Patients: Hodgkin's disease (stage II B, III B, IV A—B) and lymphoreticular sarcomas (stage II B, III A—B, IV A—B).

Treatment: Therapy consists of 6 2-week cycles with 2-week interval between each cycle. This is considered the induction phase of treatment and it takes about 6 months to complete. After 1—2 months from the sixth cycle, patients with stage II and III are subsequently irradiated (consolidation). Maintenance therapy consist of cyclophosphamide, vinblastine, procarbazine and Methotrexate given sequentially. Each drug is administered for 3 weeks. In absence of relapse, treatment is completed at the end of the third year.

marrow reserve, since leukopenia and thrombocytopenia, though reversible, almost invariably occur after one or two cycles. Sequential chemotherapy, on the other hand, can be administered in most cases on an ambulatory basis. A number of studies have demonstrated that adequate courses of chemotherapy can prolong survival in responsive patients with malignant lymphomas [101]. Since the recent results of combination chemotherapy have shown that long-term remissions can also be achieved, it is of great importance to plan a proper treatment of malignant lymphomas in the far advanced stages, too.

6. Conclusions

Malignant lymphomas, and particularly Hodgkin's disease, have received increasing attention during the past decade. Despite progress in their natural history, diagnostic evaluation and therapeutic management, their cause remains a mystery. The frequent association in Hodgkin's disease of herpes zoster [118] and the occasional concurrence with leukoencephalopathy [31] suggest a viral origin, although an infective etiology has still to be proved. The most important results achieved in the last decade are related to increased survival after radiation therapy in localized disease, thus proving that the lymphoma can be unicentric in origin, and after chemotherapy in more advanced stages. Cure is possible with a properly planned intensive irradiation and a more optimistic and aggressive approach at all stages of the disease is strongly recommended. Radiotherapists and chemotherapists should know the possibilities as well as the limits of intensive irradiation and of available drugs, respectively. They should cooperate in order to work out the most useful treatment for each case. Although several prognostic factors [8, 49, 77, 78, 82, 117, 127] are involved in malignant lymphomas, including the immunological response [1, 2, 3, 122], the single most important factor is related to the initial anatomical extent of the disease. From this point of view, although more accurate informations are expected from diagnostic laparotomy carried out in unselected large group of patients, lymphography still represents in most cases an essential step in determining the clinical stage.

References

1. Aisenberg, A. C.: Studies of lymphocyte transfer reactions in Hodgkin's disease. J. clin. Invest. **44**, 555 (1965).
2. — Immunologic status of Hodgkin's disease. Cancer **19**, 385 (1966).
3. — Manifestations of immunologic unresponsiveness in Hodgkin's disease. Cancer Res. **26**, 1152 (1966).
4. Amiel, J. L., Berumen, L., Schwartzenberg, L., Schneider, M., Cattan, A., Schlumbergher, J. R., Mathé, G.: Essai de traitment de la maladie de Hodgkin généralisée par une chimiothérapie multiple. Sem. Hôp. Paris **49**, 2970 (1966).
5. Banfi, A., Bonadonna, G., Carnevali, G., Oldini, C., Salvini, E.: Preferential sites of involvement and mode of spread in malignant lymphomas. Europ. J. Cancer **4**, 319 (1968).
6. — — — Fossati-Bellani, F.: Malignant lymphomas: further studies on their preferential sites of involvement and possible mode of spread. Lymphology **2**, 130 (1969).
7. — — — Molinari, R., Monfardini, S., Salvini, E.: Lymphoreticular sarcomas with primary onset in the Waldeyer's ring (clinical evaluation of 225 cases). Cancer **26**, 341 (1970).
8. Bennett, J. M., Nathanson, L., Rutenburg, A. M.: Significance of leukocyte alkaline phosphatase in Hodgkin's disease. Arch. intern. Med. **121**, 338 (1968).
9. Bernard, J., Boiron, M., Goguel, A., Jacquillat, C., Janzer, J., Weil, M.: Traitement de la maladie de Hodgkin par une polychimiothérapie associant moutarde à l'azote, vincristine, méthylhydrazine et prednisone. Presse méd. **75**, 2647 (1967).
10. — Jacquillat, C., Boiron, M., Weil, M., Soto, R.: Traitement de la maladie de Hodgkin par vincaleukoblastine. Presse méd. **72**, 1471 (1964).
11. Bilgutay, A. M. et al.: Mediastinoscopy. J. thorac. cardiovasc. Surg. **57**, 811 (1969).
12. Bleehen, N. M., Jeliffe, A. M.: Vinblastine sulfate in the treatment of malignant disease. Brit. J. Cancer **19**, 268 (1965).
13. Bonadonna, G., Banfi, A., Carnevali, G., Milani, F., Salvini, E.: Preferential sites and mode of spread of Hodgkin's disease and lymphoreticular sarcomas on the basis of clinical evaluation of 500 cases. Tumori **53**, 551 (1967).
14. — Fossati-Bellani, F.: The spread of malignant lymphomas in children. Tumori **54**, 311 (1968).
15. — Monfardini, S., Guindani, A.: Daunomycin treatment in chronic lymphoproliferative disorders. Tumori **54**, 465 (1968).
16. — — Oldini, C.: Comparative effects of vinblastine and procarbazine in advanced Hodgkin's disease. Europ. J. Cancer **5**, 393 (1969).
17. — — de Lena, M., Fossati-Bellani, F.: Clinical evaluation of adriamycin, a new antitumor antibiotic. Brit. med. J. **3**, 503 (1969).
18. — — Phase I and preliminary phase II evaluation of adriamycin (NSC 49842). Cancer Res. **30**, 2572 (1970).

18a. Bonadonna, G., de Lena, M., Bartoli, C., Bajetta, E., Beretta, G., Molinari, R., Guzzon, A., Fossati-Bellani, F., Monfardini, S.: Clinical trial with bleomycin in lymphomas and solid tumors. Proc. Am. Ass. Cancer Res. **12**, 11 (1971).

19. BOURONCLE, G. A.: Sternberg-Reed cells in the peripheral blood of patients with Hodgkin's disease. Blood **27,** 544 (1966).
20. BRUNNER, K. W., YOUNG, C. W.: A methylhydrazine derivative in Hodgkin's disease and other malignant neoplasms (therapeutic and toxic effects studied in 51 patients). Ann. intern. Med. **63,** 69 (1965).
21. BURCH, G. E. et al.: Effects of radiation on the human heart. Arch. intern. Med. **121,** 230 (1968).
22. CAHN, E. L., STEINFELD, J. L. (Eds.): Conference on lymphography (Bethesda 12—13 January 1967). Cancer Chemother. Rep. **52,** 1 (1968).
23. CARBONE, P. P., SPURR, C. (Chairmen): Management of patients with malignant lymphoma: a comparative study with cyclophosphamide and vinca alkaloyds. Cancer Res. **28,** 811 (1968).
24. CARNEVALI, G., SALVINI, E.: Results of radiotherapy in 144 cases of lymphosarcomas and reticulum cell sarcoma with primary onset in the pharynx. Tumori **54,** 135 (1968).
25. CATLIN, D.: Surgery for head and neck lymphomas. Surgery **60,** 1060 (1966).
25a. Clinical screening Co-operative group of the European Organization for Research on the Treatment of Cancer: Study of the clinical efficiency of bleomycin in human cancer. Brit. med. J. **1970 II,** 643.
26. COOK, J. C., KRABBNHOFT, K. L., LEUCUTIA, T.: Combined radiation and nitrogen mustard therapy in Hodgkin's disease as compared with radiation therapy alone. Amer. J. Roentgenol. **82,** 651 (1959).
27. COHN, STEWART, FAYARDO, HANCOK: Heart disease following radiation. Medicine **46,** 281 (1967).
28. Cooperative Study: Neoplastic disease. Treatment with vinblastine. Arch. intern. Med. **116,** 846 (1965).
29. CROSS, R. M.: A clinicopathological study of nodular sclerosing in Hodgkin's disease. J. clin. Path. **21,** 303 (1968).
30. DAMASCELLI, B., BONADONNA, G., MUSUMECI, R., USLENGHI, C.: Two-dimensional pulsed echo detection of para-aortic lymph nodes. Surg. Gynec. Obstet. **128,** 772 (1969).
31. DEEP, W. D., FRAUMENI, J. F., TASHIMA, C. K., MC DAVITT, R.: Leukoencephalopathy and dermatomyositis in Hodgkin's disease. Arch. intern. Med. **113,** 635 (1964).
32. DEVITA, V. T., SERPICK, A.: Combination chemotherapy in the treatment of Hodgkin's disease.
33. — — CARBONE, P. P.: Combination chemotherapy of advanced Hodgkin's disease. Proc. Amer. Ass. Cancer Res. **10,** 19 (1969).
34. DI PIETRO, S., PIZZETTI, F.: Histology as a prognostic factor in 100 cases of Hodgkin's disease. Tumori **52,** 451 (1967).
35. EASSON, E. C., RUSSEL, M. H.: The cure of Hodgkin's disease. Brit. med. J. **1963 I,** 1704.
36. — Radiotherapy for malignant lymphomas. Ann. Rev. Med. **17,** 179 (1966).
37. EHRLICH, A. N., STALDER, G., GELLER, W., SHERLOCK, P.: Gastrointestinal manifestations of malignant lymphoma. Gastroenterology **54,** 1115 (1968).
38. ENGEST, A., BRENNHOUD, I. O., CHRISTENSEN, I., HAGEN, S., HOEG, S., HOST, H., LIVERUD, K., NESHEIM, A.: Sternberg-Reed cells in the thoracic duct lymph of patients with Hodgkin's disease. Blood **31,** 99 (1968).
39. EZDINLI, E. Z., STUTZMAN, L.: Vinblastine versus nitrogen mustard therapy of Hodgkin's disease. Cancer **22,** 473 (1968).
40. FAIRLEY, G. H., PATTERSON, M. J. L., SCOTT, R. B.: Chemotherapy of Hodgkin's disease with cyclophosphamide, vinblastine and procarbazine. Brit. med. J. **1966 II,** 75.
41. FLATOW, F. A., ULTMAN, J. E., HYMAN, G. A., MUGGIA, F. M.: Treatment of advanced Hodgkin's disease with vinblastine (NSC - 49842) or procarbazine (NSC - 77213). Cancer Chemother. Rep. **53,** 39 (1969).
42. FORCIER, R. Y., MCINTYRE, O. R.: Combination chemotherapy of advanced lymphoma. Cancer Chemother. Rep. **53,** 86 (1969).
43. FRANSSILA, K. O., KALIMA, T. V., VOUTILAINEN, A.: Histologic classification of Hodgkin's disease. Cancer **20,** 1954 (1967).

44. Frei III, E., deVita, V. T., Moxley III, J. H., Carbone, P. P.: Approaches to improving the chemotherapy of Hodgkin's disease. Cancer Res. **26**, 1284 (1966).
45. — and Gamble, J. F.: Progress in the chemotherapy of Hodgkin's disease. Cancer **19**, 378 (1966).
46. Fuller, L. M., Fletcher, G. H.: The radiotherapeutic management of the lymphomatous diseases. Amer. J. Roentgenol. **88**, 909 (1962).
47. Grace, J. T., Jr., Mittleman, A.: Surgery in the management of Hodgkin's disease. Cancer **19**, 351 (1966).
48. Glenn, D. W., Faw, F. L., Kagan, A. R., Johnson, R. E.: Field reparation in multiple portal radiation therapy. Amer. J. Roentgenol. **52**, 199 (1968).
49. Gordon, H. W., Wilson, W. W., Beutler, E.: Response of the fever of Hodgkin's disease to nitrogen mustard (NSC - 762); an evaluation of its significance. Cancer Chemother. Rep. **53**, 127 (1969).
50. Hall, T. C.: New chemotherapeutic agents in Hodgkin's disease. Cancer Res. **26**, 1297 (1966).
51. — Choi, O. S., Abadi, A., Krant, M. J.: High-dose corticoid therapy in Hodgkin's disease and other lymphomas. Ann. intern. Med. **66**, 1144 (1967).
52. Han, T., Stutzman, L.: Mode of spread in patients with localized malignant lymphoma. Arch. intern. Med. **120**, 1 (1967).
53. Hanson, T. A. S.: Histological classification and survival in Hodgkin's disease. Cancer **17**, 1595 (1964).
54. Hoogstraten, B. et al.: Combination chemotherapy in lymphosarcoma and reticulum cell sarcoma. Blood **33**, 370 (1969).
55. Jacobb, M. L., Marasso, F. Y.: Lymphomas: relationship between dosage and recurrence. Radiology **83**, 106 (1964).
56. Jacobs, E. M., Peters, F. C., Luce, J. K., Zippin, C., Wood, D. A.: Mechloretamine HCl and cyclophosphamide in the treatment of Hodgkin's disease and the lymphomas. J. Amer. med. Ass. **203**, 392 (1968).
57. Jeliffe, A. M.: Vinblastine in the treatment of Hodgkin's disease. Brit. J. Cancer **32**, 44 (1969).
58. Jenkin, R. D. T., Peters, M. V., Darte, Y. M. M.: Hodgkin's disease in children. Amer. J. Roentgenol. **100**, 222 (1967).
59. Johnson, R. E., Foley, H. T., Steckel, R. Y., Glenn, D. W.: Extended radiotherapy in advanced Hodgkin's disease. Arch. intern. Med. **118**, 70 (1966).
60. — — Swain, R. W., O'Connor, G. T.: Treatment of lymphosarcoma with fractionated total body irradiation. Cancer **20**, 482 (1967).
61. — Kagan, A. R., Hafermann, M. D., Keyes, J. N., Jr.: Patient tolerance to extended irradiation. Ann. intern. Med. **70**, 1 (1969).
61 a. — Thomas, L. B., Chretien, P.: Correlation between clinicohistologic staging and extranodal relapse in Hodgkin's disease. Cancer **25**, 1071 (1970).
62. Kagan, A. R., Morton, D. L., Hafermann, R. E., Johnson, R. E.: Evaluation and management of radiation induced pericardial effusion. Radiology **92**, 632 (1969).
63. Kaplan, H. S., Rosenberg, S. A.: The treatment of Hodgkin's disease. Med. Clin. N. Amer. **50**, 1591 (1966).
64. — Role of intensive radiotherapy in the management of Hodgkin's disease. Cancer **19**, 356 (1966).
65. — Rosenberg, S. A.: Extended field radical radiotherapy in advanced Hodgkin's disease: short-term results of a randomized clinical trials. Cancer Res. **26**, 1268 (1966).
66. — Long-term results of palliative and radical radiotherapy of Hodgkin's disease. Cancer Res. **26**, 1250—1252 (1966).
67. — Clinical evaluation and radiotherapeutic management of Hodgkin's disease and the malignant lymphomas. New Engl. J. Med. **278**, 892 (1968).
68. — Prognostic significance of the relapse-free interval after radiotherapy of Hodgkin's disease. Cancer **22**, 1131 (1968).
69. Karnofsky, D. A.: Chemotherapy of Hodgkin's disease. Cancer **19**, 371 (1966).
70. — Miller, D. G., Phillips, R. F.: Role of chemotherapy in the management of early Hodgkin's disease. Amer. J. Roentgenol. **40**, 968 (1963).

71. Kaung, D. T., Whittington, R. M., Spencer, H., Patno, M. E.: Comparison of chlorambucil and streptonigrin (NSC - 45383) in the treatment of malignant lymphomas. Cancer **23,** 1280 (1969).
72. Keller, A. R., Kaplan, H. S., Lukes, R. J., Rappaport, H. D.: Correlation of histopathology with other prognostic indicators in Hodgkin's disease. Cancer **22,** 477 (1969).
73. Kenis, Y.: The treatment of Hodgkin's disease by procarbazine. Brux.-méd. **48,** 447 (1968).
74. — Werli, J., Hildebrand, J., Tagnon, H. J.: Action d'un dérivé de la méthylhydrazine, le R04-6467, dans la maladie de Hodgkin, dans d'autres lymphomes malins et dans les leucémies. Europ. J. Cancer **1,** 33 (1965).
75. Lacher, M.: Long survival in Hodgkin's disease. Ann. intern. Med. **70,** 7 (1969).
76. Lacher, M. J., Durant, J. R.: Combined vinblastine and chlorambucil therapy of Hodgkin's disease. Ann. intern. Med. **62,** 468 (1965).
76 a. Lovenbraun, S., de Vita, V., Serpick, A. A.: Combination chemotherapy with nitrogen mustard, vincristine, procarbazine and prednisone in lymphosarcoma and reticulum cell sarcoma. Cancer **25,** 1018 (1970).
77. Lawler, S. D., Pentycross, C. R., Reeves, B. R.: Lymphocyte transformation and chromosome studies in Hodgkin's disease. Brit. med. J. **3,** 704 (1966).
78. Leroy, E. C., Carbone, P. P., Sjoerdsma, A.: Elevated plasma levels of an hydroxyproline — containing protein in Hodgkin's disease and their relation to disease activity. J. Lab. clin. Med. **67,** 891 (1967).
79. Lessner, H. E., BCNU 1,3,bis(B-chlorethyl)-1-nitrosourea: Effects on advanced Hodgkin's disease and other neoplasia. Cancer (Philad.) **22,** 451 (1968).
80. Lipton, A., Viola, M., Tauro, G., Gee, T., Krakoff, I., Clarkson, B.: Treatment of leukemias and lymphomas in adults with E. Coli L-Asparaginase (L-A 'Ase). Cancer Chemother. Rep. **53,** 89 (1969).
81. Loehr, W. J. et al.: Primary lymphoma of the gastrointestinal tract. A review of 100 cases. Ann. Surg. **170,** 232 (1969).
82. Lobell, M., Boggs, D. R., Wintrobe, M. M.: The clinical significance of fever in Hodgkin's disease. Arch. intern. Med. **117,** 335 (1966).
82 a. Lovenbraun, S., Ramsay, H., Sutherland, J., Serpick, A. A.: Diagnostic laparotomy and splenectomy for staging of Hodgkin's disease. Ann. int. Med. **72,** 655 (1970). (1969) **55,** 197 (1969).
83. Luce, J. K., Gamble, J. G.: Combination chemotherapy (MOPP) in disseminated Hodgkin's disease (HD). Cancer Chemother. Rep. **53,** 89 (1969).
84. Lukes, R. J., Butler, J. Y.: The pathology and the nomenclature of Hodgkin's disease. Cancer Res. **26,** 1063 (1966).
85. — — Hicks, E.: Natural history of Hodgkin's disease as related to its pathologic picture. Cancer **19,** 317 (1966).
86. Mathé, G., Berumen, L., Schweisguth, O., Brulé, G., Schneider, M., Cattan, A., Amiel, J. L., Schwarzenberg, L.: Methyl-hydrazine in treatment of Hodgkin's disease and various forms of haematosarcomas and leukaemia. Lancet **1963 II,** 1077.
87. Miller, D. G.: Chemotherapy as a primary treatment of Hodgkin's disease. Cancer Res. **26,** 1303 (1966).
88. Molander, D. W., Pack, G. T. (Editors): Hodgkin's disease. Springfield (Ill.): Charles C Thomas 1968.
89. Monfardini, S., Bonadonna, G., di Pietro, S., Guindani, A., Fossati-Bellani, F., de Lena, M.: Clinical trials of adriamycin in leukemia and solid tumors. Tumori **55,** 197 (1969).
90. Moxley, J. H. III, Vita, V. T., Brace, K., Frei III E.: Intensive combination chemotherapy and X-irradiation in Hodgkin's disease. Cancer Res. **27,** 1258 (1967).
91. Musshoff, K., Boutis, L.: Therapy results in Hodgkin's disease (Freiburg i. Br. 1948, 1966). Cancer **21,** 1110 (1968).
92. Naqui, M. S., Burrows, L., Kark, A. E.: Lymphoma of the gastrointestinal tract. Prognostic guides based on 162 cases. Ann. Surg. **170,** 221—231 (1969).
92 a. Nicholson, W. M. et al.: Combination chemotherapy in generalized Hodgkin's disease. Brit. med. J. **3,** 7 (1970).

93. Nobler, P. M.: An optimistic and aggressive approach to the treatment of malignant lymphoma. Ann. intern. Med. **68**, 414 (1968).
94. Pack, G. T., Molander, D. W.: The surgical treatment of Hodgkin's disease. Cancer Res. **26**, 1254 (1966).
95. Papaioannou, A. N., Watson, W. L.: Primary lymphoma of the lung: an appraisal of its natural hystory and a comparison with other localized lymphomas. J. thorac. cardiovasc. Surg. **49**, 373 (1965).
96. Peters, M. V.: A study of survivals in Hodgkin's disease treated radiologically. Amer. J. Roentgenol. **63**, 956 (1950).
97. — Middlemiss, K. C. H.: A study of Hodgkin's disease treated by irradiation. Amer. J. Roentgenol. **78**, 114 (1958).
98. — The contributions of radiation therapy in the control of early lymphomas. Amer. J. Roentgenol. **90**, 956 (1963).
99. — Prophylactic treatment of adjacent areas in Hodgkin's disease. Cancer Res. **26**, 1232 (1966).
100. — Alison, R. E., Busch, R. S.: Natural history of Hodgkin's disease as related to staging. Cancer **19**, 308 (1966).
100 a. Perry, S., Thomas, L. B., Johnson, R. E., Carbone, P. P., Haynes, H. A.: Hodgkin's disease: combined clinical staff conference at the National Institutes of Health. Ann. intern. Med. **67**, 424 (1967).
101. Rapoport, A., Cole, P., Mason, J.: Correlates of Survival after initiation of chemotherapy in 142 cases of Hodgkin's disease. Cancer **24**, 377 (1969).
102. Rappaport, H., Strum, S. B.: Concerning the spread of Hodgkin's disease: the incidence and histopathologic aspects of vascular invasion as observed in biopsy section (in press).
103. Rege, V. B., Lenhard, R. E. Jr.: BCNU(1,3-bis(2-chloroethyh)-1-nitrosourea; NSC 409962). Its effectiveness and toxicologic data in the treatment of advanced Hodgkin's disease (HD), lymphosarcoma (LYS) and reticulum cell sarcoma (RCS). Cancer Chemother. Rep. **53**, 92 (1969).
104. Rivers, S. L., Whittington, R. M., Madrek, T. M.: Treatment of malignant lymphomas with methyl ester of streptonigrin (NSC-45384). Cancer (Philad.) **19**, 1377 (1966).
105. Rosenberg, S. A., Diamond, A. D., Dargeon, H. W., Graver, L. F.: Lymphosarcoma in childhood. New Engl. J. Med. **259**, 505 (1958).
106. — Report of the Committee on the staging of Hodgkin's disease. Cancer Res. **26**, 1310 (1966).
107. — Kaplan, H. S.: Evidence for an orderly progression in the spread of Hodgkin's disease. Cancer Res. **26**, 1225 (1966).
108. Rubin, P., Kurohara, S. S.: Has prophylactic irradiation proved itself in the treatment of localized Hodgkin's disease? Radiology **87**, 240 (1966).
109. Samuels, M. L., Leary, M. V., Alexanian, R., Howe, C. D., Frei III, E.: Clinical trials with N-isoproyl-a(2-methylhydrazino)-P-toluamide hydrochloride in malignant lymphoma and other disseminated neoplasia. Cancer (Philad.) **20**, 1187 (1967).
110. Scheer, A. C.: The course of stage I malignant lymphomas following local treatment. Amer. J. Roentgenol. **90**, 939 (1963).
111. Scott, T. C.: The effect of nitrogen mustard and maintenance chlorambucil in the treatment of advanced Hodgkin's disease. Cancer Chemother. Rep. **27**, 27 (1963).
112. Serpick, A., Lowenbraun, S., DeVita, V. T.: Combination chemotherapy of lymphosarcoma (LSA) and reticulum cell sarcoma (RCS). Proc. Amer. Ass. Cancer Res. **10**, 78 (1969).
113. Seydel, H. G., Bloedorn, F. G., Wizenberg, M. J.: Time-dose-volume relationship in Hodgkin's disease. Radiology **89**, 919 (1967).
114. Smith, D. F., Klopp, C. T.: The value of surgical removal of localized lymphomas. Surgery **49**, 469 (1961).
115. Smithers, D. W.: Hodgkin's disease. Brit. med. J. **1967 II**, 263 and 337.
116. Sohier, W. D., Wong, R. K. L., Aisenberg, A. C.: Vinblastine in the treatment of advanced Hodgkin's disease. Cancer **22**, 467 (1968).

117. Sokal, J. E., Aungst, W. C.: Response to BCG vaccination and survival in advance Hodgkin's disease. Cancer **23**, 128—134 (1969).
118. — Firat, D.: Varicella — zoster infection in Hodgkin's disease: clinical and epidemiological aspects. Amer. J. Med. **39**, 452, 463 (1965).
119. Stephenson, P. A., Lee, B. J.: Prognostic and therapeutic implications of the lymphangiogram in Hodgkin's disease. Cancer Chemother. Rep. **53**, 94 (1969).
120. Storti, E.: Peut — on considérer la lymphogranulomatose comme une maladie à debut localisé? Nécessité d'un diagnostic précoce. Bull. Mém. Soc. Med. Paris (n⁰ 16, Seance du 27 Novembre 1937).
121. Stutzam, L.: Simultaneous vs. sequential multiple agent chemotherapy of Hodgkin's disease. Cancer Chemother. Rep. **53**, 95 (1969).
122. Svet-Moldavsky, G. J.: Is Hodgkin's disease a syndrome of hypothymism? Nature **209**, 932 (1966).
123. *Symposium international „la radiotherapie de la maladie de Hodgkin"* (Paris, 15 Février 1965). Nouv. Rev. franç. Hémat. **6**, 7 (1966).
124. *Symposium on clinical aspects of Hodgkin's disease* (New York, November 22, 1965). Cancer **19**, 297 (1966).
125. *Symposium on obstacles to the control of Hodgkin's disease* (Rye, N. Y. 13—15 September 1965). Cancer Res. **26**, 1046 (1966).
126. Todd, I. D. H.: Natulan in the management of late Hodgkin's disease, other lymphoreticular sarcomas, and malignant melanoma. Brit. med. J. **1965 II**, 628.
127. Trubowitz, S., Masek, B., del Rosario, A.: Lymphocyte response to phytohemagglutinin in Hodgkin's disease, lymphatic leukemia and lymphosarcoma. Cancer **19**, 2019 (1966).
128. van der Werf-Messing, B.: Reticulum cell sarcoma and Lymphosarcoma. A retrospective study of potential survival in loco-regional disease. Europ. J. Cancer **4**, 549 (1968).
129. Vogel, J. M., Kimball, H. R., Foley, H. T., Wolff, S. M., Perry, S.: The effect of extensive radiotherapy on the marrow granulocyte reserves of patients with Hodgkin's disease. Cancer **21**, 798 (1968).
130. Williams, H. M., Diamond, H. D., Craver, L. F.: The pathogenesis and management of neurological complications in patients with malignant lymphomas and leukemia. Cancer **11**, 75 (1958).
131. Yount, W. J., Finkel, H. E.: Treatment of refractory reticulum cell sarcoma with low doses of vincristine sulfate. J. Amer. med. Ass. **197**, 535 (1966).

Chapter 2

Lymphangiography and Endolymphatic Radiotherapy: General Principles

S. Chiappa, R. Musumeci, and C. Uslenghi

With 3 Figures

In 1952 the technique of direct lymphography, as an elective method of exploration and study of the peripheral lymphatic collectors and of the lymph nodes located along the peripheral lymphatic ways, was first studied and tested in clinical practice by J. B. Kinmonth [46—48]. Since then, the use of lymphography as a diagnostic tool has spread and been adopted in all countries and there have been very many contributions to the literature on the subject from various research groups [1, 5, 6, 8, 10—11, 13—15, 23, 25—30, 34—43, 49—61, 67—72, 76, 78—84, 86—88]. Numerous investigators in many countries authoritatively state that lymphographic reports are very reliable, especially in the field of lymphoproliferative diseases [6, 8, 10, 15, 23, 25, 27, 29, 37—38, 40, 43, 49, 52, 54—55, 57, 61, 67, 78—79, 84, 86—88].

In the field of the so-called malignant lymphomas, lymphography has therefore made a valuable contribution both to our knowledge of the mode of spread of these diseases, and to the planning of adequate programs for treatment. In the light of modern trends of radiotherapy in malignant lymphomas, it is evident that a classification by stages is of vital importance. This classification should not be based only on the empiric findings of indirect X-ray and physical examinations, but on an objective and accurate demonstration of the lymph-node groups involved [8—9, 24—25, 27, 29, 37—38, 43, 54—55, 61, 83, 87—88].

The possibility of gaining direct access to the lymphatics of the lower extremities suggested the idea of utilizing this technique to provide an elective tissue therapy which would spare the neighbouring tissues and the body in general as much as possible. Lymphography offers two possibilities to those who deal with these problems in the field of cancer research: the administration through the lymphatics of anticancer drugs and of radioactive isotopes. Among the chemotherapeutic agents, we would mention cyclophosphamine, mechlorethamine, Methotrexate, 5-fluorouracil, etc. [2, 18—20].

With regard to radio-isotopes, the introduction of radionuclides into the lymphatic system has been proposed and carried out in experimental animals as well as in man, especially with ^{198}Au, for a topographical exploration of the lymph centres [31—32, 73]. The introduction of radioisotopes into the lymphatic system exclusively for therapeutic purposes was carried out for the first time in September 1961 by S. CHIAPPA et al. in our Institute, using as the radioactive agent the iodine of the oily contrast material employed for diagnostic investigation (Lipiodol F or UF), substituted in part by its isotope ^{131}I.

This new method of internal irradiation, which differs from the traditional criteria of external antineoplastic radiotherapy, has been called "*endolymphatic radiotherapy*" (E.R.T.) [14—24, 62—65].

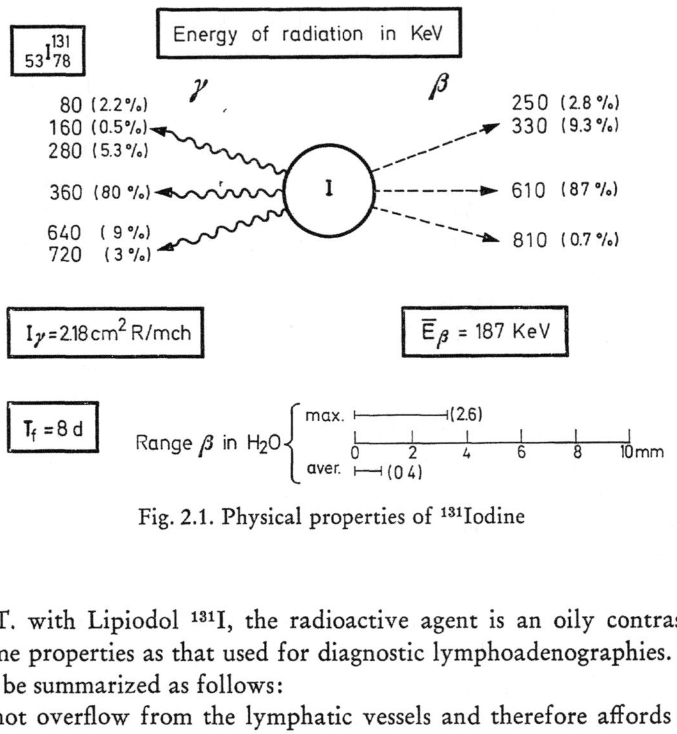

Fig. 2.1. Physical properties of ^{131}Iodine

In E.R.T. with Lipiodol ^{131}I, the radioactive agent is an oily contrast material with the same properties as that used for diagnostic lymphoadenographies. Its characteristics can be summarized as follows:

it does not overflow from the lymphatic vessels and therefore affords reasonable safety in usage;

it visualizes an extensive lymphatic area;

it opacifies the lymph nodes it reaches to an equal extent, provided the marginal sinus of the lymph node has the same permeability;

it remains in the lymph nodes for a relatively long time (an average of 8—10 months). The fact that it remains within the lymph nodes enables us to make an objective radiographic evaluation of the size of the lymph nodes over a period of time, and therefore of both growth and shrinkage.

We should now examine the reasons why we prefer to use ^{131}I rather than other radioactive substances. Figs. 2.1, 2.2, and 2.3 show the most important physical properties of some isotopes commonly used in endolymphatic radiotherapy (^{131}I,

^{198}Au, ^{32}P). ^{131}I has some very favourable characteristics that can be summarized as follows:

it has a half-life of 8 days;

its emission of β radiations is sufficiently powerful (87% of 610 KeV and 12.3% of about 300 KeV);

its emission of γ radiations enables us to view the material introduced from outside (scintiscan);

the radioactive material remains in the lymph nodes because it forms a stable bond with a carrier molecule which is electively lymphotrophic.

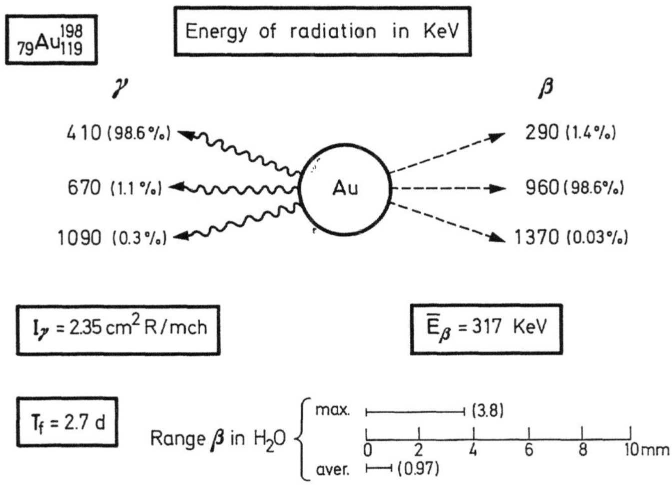

Fig. 2.2. Physical properties of ^{198}Gold

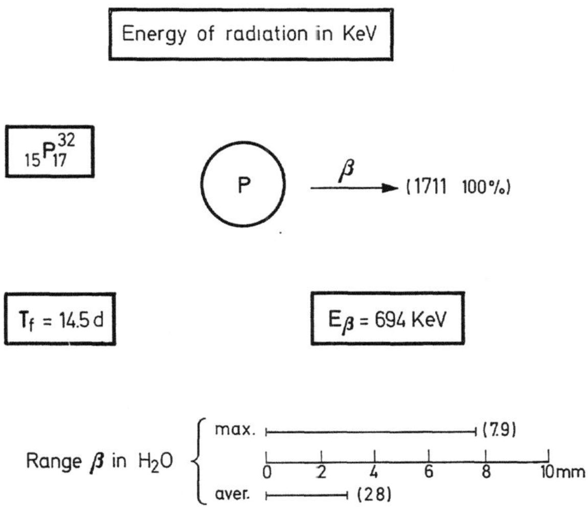

Fig. 2.3. Physical properties of ^{32}Phosphorus

The characteristics of ^{131}I also enable us to make an accurate study of its distribution and metabolism in the body. With ^{32}P a scintiscan study is not always possible or easy, as this is a pure β-emitting substance. We should also consider the possibility of hematopoietic damage, as phosphorus tends to accumulate in the bone marrow where it has a high turnover. Recent clinical observations [4] on the use of ceramic microspheres activated with ^{90}Y seem to have given promising results [3—4, 7, 12, 31—32, 73]. In 1964 SEITZMAN et al. [75] published a report on the use of Ethiodol ^{131}I, an iodized oil with physical and chemical properties similar to those of Lipiodol UF. This radioactive contrast material is that predominantly used in the U.S.A.

Table 2.1. *Authors who employed E.R.T. are listed with the year and the radionuclide used*

Author	Year	Radionuclide
RATTI and CHIAPPA	1962	^{131}I
ARIEL	1963	^{131}I
SEITZMAN et al.	1963	^{131}I
OMNIS et al.	1963	^{131}I
PICARD et al.	1964	^{131}I
ARIEL	1964	^{90}Y
ARIEL	1964	^{198}Au
LAMARQUE et al.	1964	^{131}I
BURGER	1964	^{32}P
LIEBNER	1965	^{131}I
FISHER	1965	^{131}I
VECCHIETTI et al.	1965	^{32}P
TILAK et al.	1966	^{131}I
EDWARDS	1966	^{131}I
RYZICK	1966	^{131}I
and many others.		

The radio-opacity and γ emission of Lipiodol ^{131}I permit the evaluation of its fundamental properties when therapeutic action takes place, namely the accumulation of the radionuclide in the area involved, whether it remains there long enough to provide adequate irradiation, and whether it is satisfactorily distributed between the involved area and neighbouring tissues or organs. The theoretical concept behind this new method of radiotherapy is, therefore, to administer very high tissue-doses, thus sparing the peripheral tissues surrounding the lymph nodes to a greater extent. In this manner a small dose-volume is administered. In the light of our own experience and that of other investigators, we feel that this objective has been achieved.

Irradiation of the lymph nodes takes place internally, obviously sparing the perilymphatic connective tissues and the organs adject to the lymph node areas. It is probably also on account of this that we have not generally local or other side-effects in the large majority of our patients. The lymph nodes are irradiated in a continuous manner, though in decreasing doses. It is also possible that the irradiation dose to the neoplastic tissues will decrease with time to a lesser extent than normally occurs for the nuclide being used. In fact, the volume in which the contrast material collects becomes gradually smaller as the lymph node shrinks. In this way, lymphnode groups spread over large areas are treated simultaneously and rapidly, since treatment is given through a single injection.

After the first clinical-therapeutic experience of CHIAPPA et al., numerous articles by both Italian and foreign authors appeared in the literature on the subject of E.R.T. This new method of radiotherapy has been evaluated and considered in various ways in the light of the therapeutic program for malignant lymphomas, but the discussion has aroused tremendous interest among those concerned with the treatment of these illnesses (Table 2.1) [2—4, 7, 9, 12, 14, 16—22, 24, 31, 33, 44, 62—66, 74—75, 77, 85, 89].

References

1. ABRAMS, H. L., TAKAHASHI, M., ADAMS, D. F.: Usefulness and accuracy of lymphangiography in lymphoma. Cancer Chemother. Rep. **52**, 157 (1968).
2. ARIEL, I. M., RESNICK, M. I.: The intralymphatic administration of radioactive isotopes and cancer-chemotherapeutic drugs. Surgery **55**, 355 (1964).
3. — — OROPEZA, R.: The intralymphatic administration of radioactive isotopes for treating malignant melanoma. Surg. Gynec. Obstet. **124**, 25 (1967).
4. — Lymphography and endolymphatic administration of radioactive isotopes for treating cancer. N.Y. St. J. Med. **68**, 1247 (1968).
5. ARVAY, N., PICARD, J. D.: La lymphographie. Etude radiologique et clinique des voies lymphatiques. Paris: Masson & Cie 1963.
6. BELTZ, L., THURN, P.: Zur Verlaufskontrolle des Lymphadenogramms bei retroperitonealen Lymphknotentumoren. Fortschr. Röntgenstr. **104**, 1 (1966).
7. BERG, H. F., CHRISTOPHERSEN, W. H.: Selective irradiation of lymph nodes by interstitial injection of radioactive colloidal gold. Amer. J. Surg. **22**, 172 (1956).
8. BISMUTH, V., BOURDON, R., DESPREZ-CURELY, J. P., MARKOVITS, P.: Lymphography in malignant Lymphomas, Panel-discussion IV. In: Progress in lymphology. Ed.: A. Ruttimann. Stuttgart: Thieme 1967, p. 160.
9. BONADONNA, G., CHIAPPA, S., MUSUMECI, R., USLENGHI, C.: Endolymphatic radiotherapy in malignant lymphomas. A clinical evaluation of 285 patients. Cancer **22**, 885 (1968).
10. BRICKNER, T. J., BOYER, C. W., PERRY, R. H.: Limited value of lymphangiography in Hodgkin's disease. Radiology **90**, 52 (1968).
11. BRUUN, S., ENGESET, A.: Lymphadenography. A new method for the visualization of enlarged lymph nodes and lymphatic vessels. Acta radiol. (Stockh.) **45**, 389 (1956).
12. BURGER, R. H.: Lymph node response to high-dose intralymphatic injection of radiochromic phosphate. Bull. N.Y. Acad. Med. **40**, 142 (1964).
13. CAVALOT, A., FARINET, G., FRANCIA, A.: Considerazioni in tema di linfografia. Minerva med. **51**, 136 (1960).
14. CHIAPPA, S.: Il valore diagnostico e terapeutico dell'adenolinfografia. Atti Accad. med. lombarda **17**, 6 (1962).
15. — GALLI, G., BARBAINI, S., RAVASI, G.: La linfografia nelle neoplasie primitive e secondarie del sistema linfoghiandolare. Radiol. Med. **48**, 1155 (1962).
16. — — — — La radioterapia endo-linfatica: primi risultati di una nuova metodica. Radiol. Med. **48**, 663 (1962).
17. — — — — La radioterapia endo-linfatica: primi risultati di una nuova metodica. Nota I: Tumori **48**, 147 (1962).
18. — — PALMIA, G.: Observations on intralymphatic radiotherapy and general chemotherapy. Clin. Radiology **15**, 202 (1964).
19. — — Considerazioni critiche sui più recenti metodi di terapia per via linfatica. Rass. clin.-sci. Ist. biochim. tal. **39**, 3 (1963).
20. — — CHIAPPA, L.: La radioterapia endolinfatica nell trattamento delle linforeticulopatie sistemiche. J. Belge Radiol. **47**, 657 (1964).

21. Chiappa, S., Galli, G., Severini, A.: Lymphadenography with radioactive contrast medium in retroperitoneal localisations of malignant lymphogranuloma. Amer. J. Roentgenol. **92**, 134 (1964).
22. — — Palmia, C., Severini, S.: Lymphography with radioactive contrast medium in lymphosarcoma and reticulosarcoma. Brit. J. Haemat. **11**, 32 (1965).
23. — Bonadonna, G., Uslenghi, C.: Lymphangiographic diagnosis of malignant lymphoma. Amer. J. Med. **40**, 290 (1966).
24. — Uslenghi, C., Bonadonna, G., Musumeci, R.: Endolymphatic radiotherapy in malignant lymphomas. Long-term results. Lymphology **3**, 13 (1970).
25. Cook, P. L., Jelliffe, A. M., Kendall, B., McLoughlin, M. J.: The role of lymphography in the diagnosis and management of malignant reticuloses. Brit. J. Radiol. **39**, 561 (1966).
26. Davidson, J. W.: Lymphography in malignant disease: Radiological aspects. Canad. med. Ass. J. **97**, 1283 (1967).
27. — Saini, M., Peters, M. V.: Lymphography in lymphoma. With particular reference to Hodgkin's disease. Radiology **88**, 281 (1967).
28. del Buono, M.: Semeiotica linfografica nelle affezioni neoplastiche. Atti XXII Congr. Naz. S.I.R.M.N. Catania 1963, vol. III, pag. 158.
29. Desprez-Curely, J. P., Bourdon, R., Bismuth, V., Bernard, J., Markovits, P.: Extension of malignant lymphoma to deep-lying lymph nodes. In: Progress in lymphology. Ed.: A. Ruttimann. Stuttgart: Thieme 1967, p. 136.
30. Dolan, P. A.: Lymphography. Brit. J. Radiol. **37**, 405 (1964).
31. Farinet, G., Cavalot, A.: Adenolinfografia con oro colloidale radioattivo. (Au 198). Minerva fisioter. **4**, 282 (1959).
32. Fischer, H. W.: Intralymphatic introduction of radioactive colloids into the lymph nodes. Radiology **79**, 297 (1962).
33. — Intralymphatic therapy for lymph node metastases of carcinoma of the cervix. An analysis of the proposition and presentation of pertinent experimental data. Cancer **18**, 1059 (1965).
34. Fuchs, W. A., Ruttimann, A., del Buono, M.: Klinische Indikationen zur Lymphographie. Schweiz. med. Wschr. **79**, 755 (1959).
35. — Book-Henderstrom, G.: Inguinal and pelvic lymphography. A preliminary report. Acta Radiol. **56**, 340 (1961).
36. — Lymphographie und Tumordiagnostik. Berlin-Heidelberg-New York: Springer 1965.
37. Hartel, M.: Prognosis of Hodgkin's disease according to radiographic pattern of lymph nodes. II international Congress of lymphology. Miami Beach 1968.
38. — — Die Prognose des Morbus Hodgkin auf Grund der Lymphknotenstruktur im Lymphogramm. Fortschr. Röntgenstr. **109**, 553 (1968).
39. Gergely, R.: The roentgen examination of the lymphatic in man. Radiology **71**, 59 (1968).
40. Hreshchysyn, M. M., Sheean, F. R.: Lymphangiography in patients with pelvic cancer and lymphomas. Proc. Amer. Ass. Cancer. Res. **3**, 121 (1960).
41. — — Holland, J. F.: Visualization of retroperitoneal lymph-nodes. Lymphangiography as an aid in the measurement of the growth tumor. Cancer **14**, 205 (1961).
42. Jackson, L. G., Wallace, S., Schaffer, R. B., Gould, J., Kramer, S., Weiss, A. J.: Diagnostic value of lymphangiography. Ann. intern. Med. **54**, 870 (1961).
43. Jing, B. S., McGraw, J. P.: Lymphangiography in diagnosis and management of malignant lymphomas. Cancer. (Philad.) **19**, 565 (1966).
44. Jantet, G. H.: Direct intralymphatic injection of radioactive colloidal gold in the treatment of malignant diseases. Brit. J. Radiol. **35**, 962 (1962).
45. — Edwards, J. M., Gough, M. H., Kinmonth, J. B.: Endolymphatic therapy with radioactive gold for malignant melanoma. Brit. med. **1964 II**, 904.
46. Kinmonth, J. B.: Lymphangiography in man. A method of outlining lymphatic trunks at operation. Clin. Sci. **11**, 13 (1952).
47. — Taylor, G. W., Harper, R. K.: Lymphangiography. Technique for its clinical use in lower limbs. Brit. med. J. **1955 I**, 940.
48. — Lymphangiography by radiological methods. J. Fac. Radiol. (Lond.) **6**, 217 (1955).

49. Koehler, P. R.: Roentgenologic aspects of lymphoma as seen on the lymphogram. Cancer Chemother. Rep. **52**, 171 (1968).
50. — Salmon, R. B.: Lymphographic patterns in lymphoma; with emphasis on the atypical form. Radiology **87**, 623 (1966).
51. — Wohl, G. T., Schaffer, B.: Lymphoangiography — a survey of its current status. Amer. J. Roentgenol. **91**, 1216 (1964).
52. Lamarque, J. L., Ginestie, J. F., Combes, C.: La lymphographie dans le diagnostic précoce des localisations profondes au cours des hémopathies malignes. J. Méd. Montpellier **2**, 31 (1967).
53. — Pages, A., Pujol, H., Ginestie, J. F., Combes, C.: Anatomie radiologique et valeur sémiologique des images ganglionnaires en lymphographie. J. Radiol. Electrol. **48**, 253 (1967).
54. Lee, B. J.: Evaluation of the patient with lymphoma by means of lymphoangiography: comments on importance and complications. In: Progress in lymphology. Ed.: A. Ruttimann. Stuttgart: Thieme 1967, p. 127.
55. — Correlation between lymphangiography and clinical status of patients with lymphoma. Cancer Chemother. Rep. **52**, 205 (1968).
56. Macdonald, J. S., Laugier, A., Schlienger, M.: Observations on the growth of tumors in lymph nodes changing from normal to abnormal while remaining opacified after lymphography. Clin. Radiol. **19**, 120 (1968).
57. Malamos, B., Moulopoulos, S. D., Sarkas, A.: Lymphadenography: its uses in haematology. Brit. med. J. **1959 II**, 1360.
58. Malek, P.: Bases physiologiques, physiopathologiques et anatomiques de la lymphographie. IX Int. Congr. Radiol. München 1959.
59. Marchal, G., Bernard, J., Arvay, N., Bilski-Pasquier, G., Ecoiffier, J., Picard, J. D.: La lymphographie dans les adénopathies profondes. Presse méd. **69**, 2253 (1961).
60. Ottaviani, G.: Indagini radiografiche sul sistema linfatico. Arch. ital. Anat. Embriol. **28**, 38 (1930).
61. Peters, M. V., Brown, T. C., Davidson, J. W., Saxena, V. S., Saini, M.: The value of locating occult disease in the treatment of Hodgkin's disease. In: Progress in lymphology. Ed.: A. Ruttiman. Stuttgart: Thieme 1967, p. 119.
62. Ratti, A., Chiappa, S., Fava, G.: I principi e le indicazioni della terapia endolinfatica con Lipiodol marcato con ^{131}I. Minerva med. **56**, 2013 (1965).
63. — La somministrazione per la via dei linfatici di isotopi radioattivi a scopo terapeutico. Minerva med. **57**, 4440 (1966).
64. — La radioterapia endolinfatica. Atti Accad. med. lombarda **21**, 2543 (1966).
65. — Chiappa, S.: La lymphographie au lipiodol radioactif dans la maladie de Hodgkin. Nouv. Rev. franç. Hémat. **6**, 155 (1966).
66. Romieu, C., Pujol, H., Lamarque, J. L.: La lymphographie radioactive dans la thérapeutique des hémopathies malignes. Presse méd. **73**, 1797 (1965).
67. Rosenberg, S. A.: Contribution of lymphangiography to our understanding of lymphoma. Cancer Chemother. Rep. **52**, 213 (1968).
68. Rouvier, H.: Anatomy of the Human Lymphatic System. Translated: M. J. Tobias Ann Arbor (MI): Edwards Brothers Inc. 1938.
69. Rusznyak, I., Foldi, M., Szabo, G.: Lymphatic System. Translated: M. J. Tobias Ann Arbor (MI): Edwards Brothers Inc. 1938, p. 318.
70. Ruttimann, A., del Buono, M. S.: Die Lymphographie mit öligem Kontrastmittel. Fortschr. Röntgenstr. **97**, 552 (1962).
71. — Die Lymphographie. In: Ergebnisse der medizinischen Strahlenforschung, N.F., Diagnostik, Therapie, Nuklearmedizin, Biologie. Hrsg.: H. R. Schinz, R. Glauner und A. Ruttimann. Bd. I. Stuttgart: Thieme 1964, S. 248.
72. Schaffer, B., Koehler, R. P., Daniel, C. R., Wohl, G. T., Rivera, E., Meyers, W. A., Skelly, J. F.: A critical evaluation of lymphoangiography. Radiology **80**, 917 (1963).
73. Schwartz, S. I., Greenlaw, R. H., Rob, C., Rubin, P.: Intralymphatic injection of radioactive gold. A preliminary experimental report. Cancer **15**, 623 (1962).
74. Seitzman, M. D., Wright, R., Halaby, F. A., Freeman, J. H.: Radioactive lymphoangiography as a therapeutic adjunct. Amer. J. Roentgenol. **89**, 140—149 (1963).

75. SEITZMAN, D. M., MALABY, F. A., FLANAGAN, P., WRIGHT, R., FREEMAN, J. H.: Intralymphatic radioisotope therapy. Surg. Gynec. Obstet. **118**, 52 (1964).
76. SHEEHAN, R., HRESHCHYSHYN, M., LIN, R. K., LESSMANN, F. P.: The use of lymphography as a diagnostic method. Radiology **76**, 47 (1961).
77. SIEGEL, P., LIEBNER, E. J.: Intralymphatic radioactive therapy for pelvic cancer. Amer. J. Obstet. Gynec. **91**, 122 (1965).
78. TAKAHASHI, M., ABRAMS, H. L.: The accuracy of lymphangiographic diagnosis in malignant lymphoma. Radiology **89**, 448 (1967).
79. TRAPP, P., FEINDT, H. R.: Zur Differentialdiagnose der malignen Lymphome aus dem Lymphogram. Fortschr. Röntgenstr. **107**, 336 (1967).
80. VIAMONTE, M. JR., ALTMAN, D., PARKS, R., BLUM, E., BEVILLACQUA, M., RECHER, L.: Radiographic-pathologic correlation in the interpretation of lymphangioadenograms. Radiology **80**, 903 (1963).
81. WALLACE, S., JACKSON, L., DODD, G. D., GREENING, R. R.: Lymphangiographic interpretation. Radiol. Clin. N. Amer. **3**, 467 (1965).
82. — — GREENING, R. R.: Clinical applications of lymphography. Amer. J. Roentgenol. **91**, 1187 (1964).
83. — —SCHAFFER, B., GOULD, J., GREENING, R. R., WEISS, A., KRAMER, S.: Lymphangiograms: their diagnostic and therapeutic potential. Radiology **76**, 179 (1961).
84. WEISSLEDER, H.: Retroperitoneale Lymphknotenveränderungen beim Morbus Hodgkin. Fortschr. Röntgenstr. **101**, 450 (1964).
85. — PFANNENSTIEL, P., STRICKSTROCK, H. K., HOFFMANN, G.: Die endolymphatische Therapie mit radioaktiven Substanzen. Fortschr. Röntgenstr. **107**, 758—764 (1967).
86. WILJASALO, M.: Lymphographic differential diagnosis of neoplastic disease. Acta radiol. (Stockh.) Suppl. **247** (1965).
87. — Lymphangiographic polymorphism in Hodgkin's disease. Acta radiol. (Stockh.) Suppl. **289** (1969).
88. WILJASALO, S.: The many lymphographic patterns of Hodgkin's disease. II International congress of Lymphology. Miami Beach 1968.
89. ZUM WINKEL, K., BECKER, J., JAHNS, E., SCHEURLEN, H., HERZFELD, U.: Indicationsstellung und Dosimetrie bei der endolymphatischen Therapie mit ^{131}A Lipiodol. Strahlentherapie **133**, 481—498 (1967).

Chapter 3

Technique of Lymphography and Endolymphatic Radiotherapy

BRUNO DAMASCELLI

With 7 Figures

The techniques used for lymphatic vessel cannulation are many but we can say that almost every investigator uses, with personal modifications, the method originally proposed by J. B. KINMONTH [1—10, 12—16, 19—20, 22—37, 39—44, 46—53].

For lymphography and E.R.T. procedures we employ specially designed needles and clamps, and an automatic electric injector [7].

Visualization of the lymphatic vessels is obtained by injection of a 1% solution of Patent Blue Violet. The injection is given in the first space between the toes and the quantity of dye used is approximately 0.5 ml for each side. Then, on the

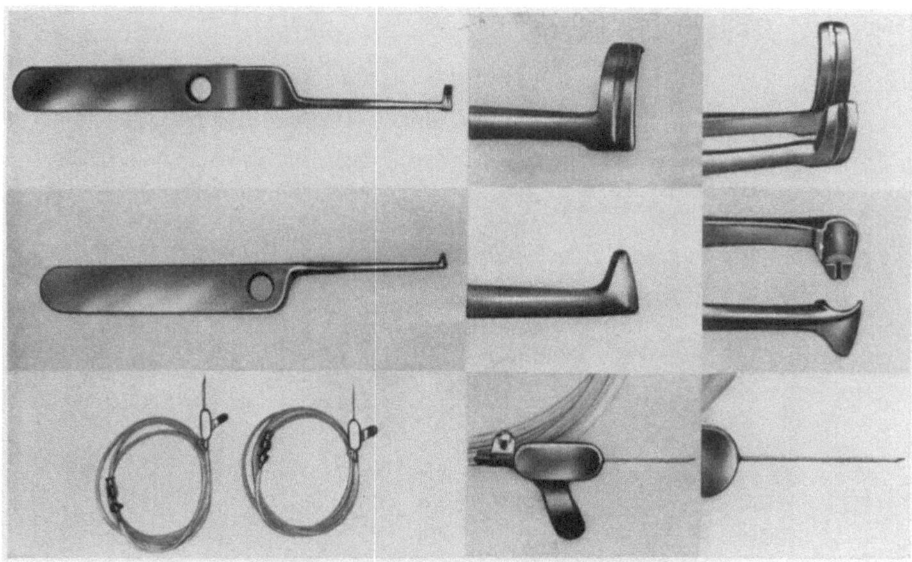

Figs. 3.1 to 3.6. See text. (By courtesy of Lymphology, 1969)

basis of definite anatomical findings, we make a longitudinal incision about 2 cm. long in the first intermetatarsal space. At this site one or more lymphatic vessels with a suitable calibre of cannulation can almost always be found.

Figs. 3.1 to 3.7 show the instruments and the procedure we use [17]. Fig. 3.1 illustrates the instruments we usually employ when performing lymphography. Fig. 3.2 is an enlarged view of the lymphatic vessel as seen after longitudinal incision of the skin. With the aid of forceps the lymphatic vessel is separated from its tunica adventitia (Fig. 3.3). A special clamp (Fig. 3.4) is used to hold the cleaned vessel.

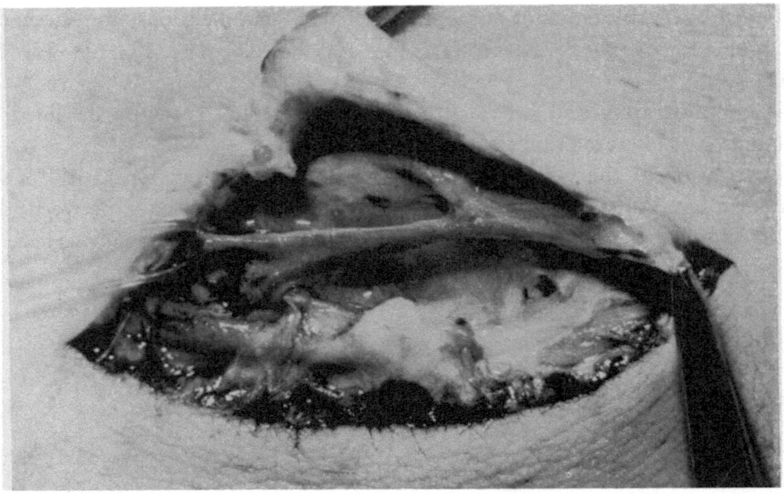

Fig. 3.2

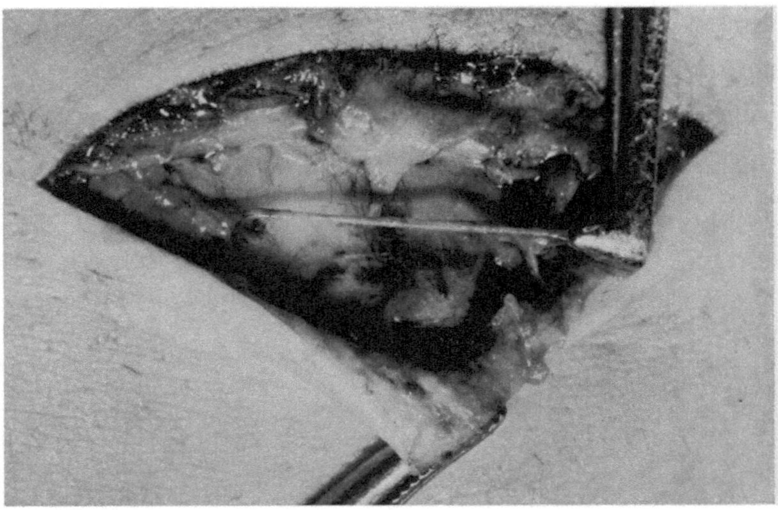

Fig. 3.3

The clamp has a groove running along both jaws; the inside of the upper jaw has small teeth that grip the lymphatic vessel. The cone-shaped tip of the forceps also has a groove along which the vessel runs and the end of the groove is a cylindrical chamber to collect the adventitial tissue that is removed when the cone runs along the vessel in a caudal direction.

The flattened needles are mounted by special grips onto a polyethylene tube. The needle has a side plate with an anatomic curve which is convenient to hold when cannulating.

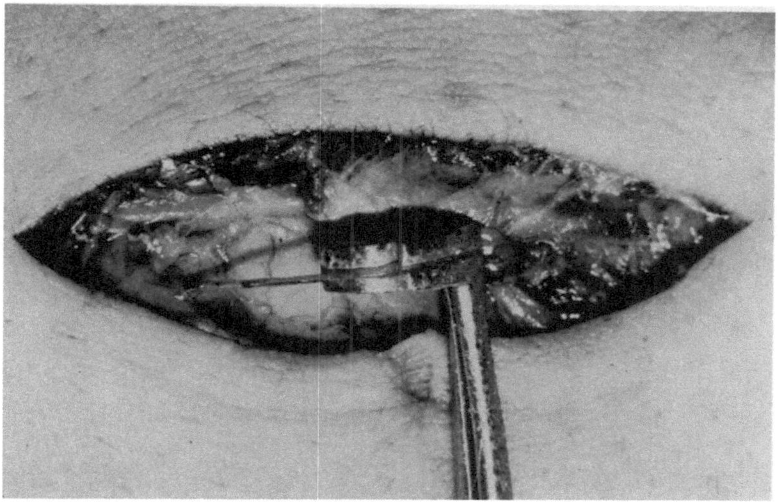

Fig. 3.4

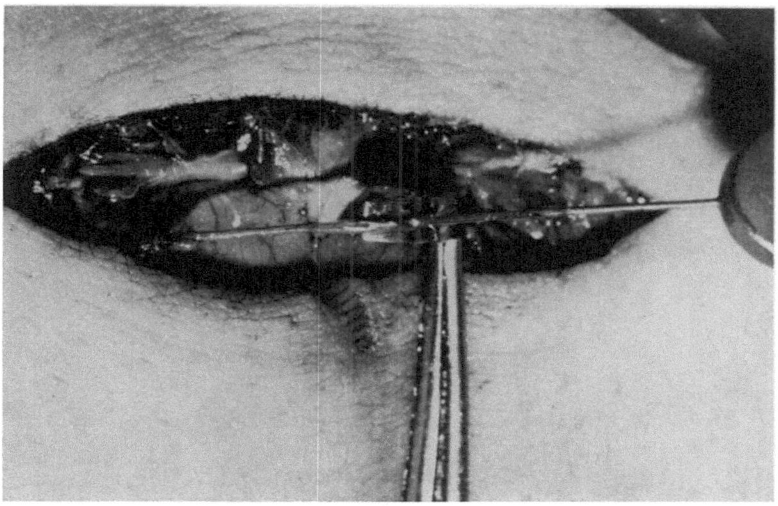

Fig. 3.5

Figs. 3.5 and 3.6 show the cannulation technique. The forceps is rotated upwards and the needle runs along the upper inlet to enter the lymph vessel. The needle is then tightly tied into position with a catgut knot and a strip of plaster.

Fig. 3.7 shows the Mayo electric constant-speed automatic injector. During the whole cannulation procedure, non-radioactive Lipiodol is used. A small plastic tube

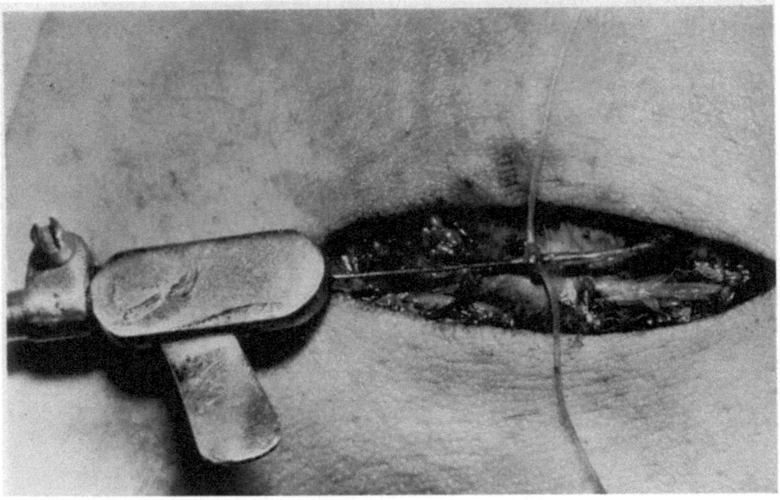

Fig. 3.6

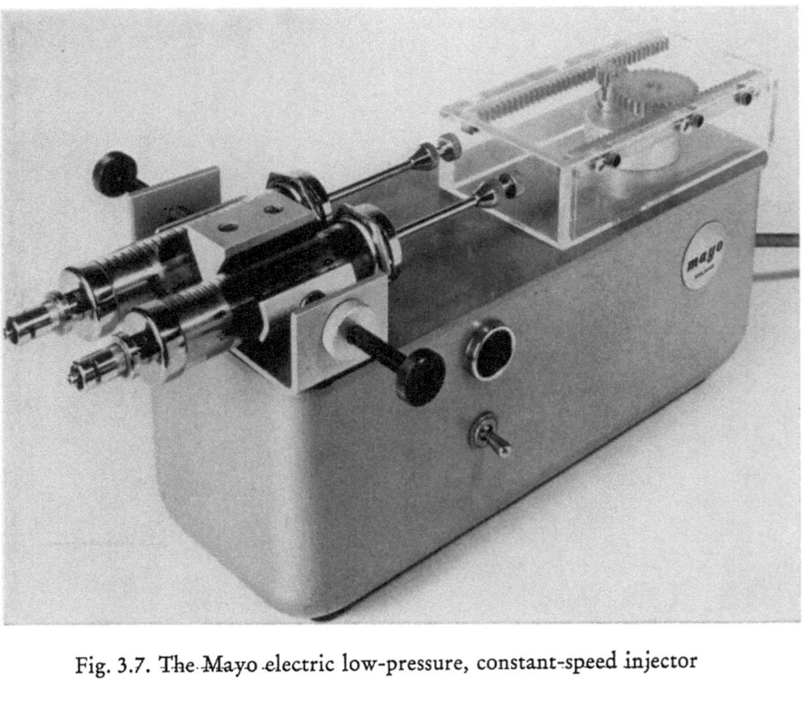

Fig. 3.7. The Mayo electric low-pressure, constant-speed injector

connecting both syringe and needle, and having a luer-lock at its free ends, is then applied to the needle.

The syringes containing the radioactive contrast material are brought to the ward where the procedure is being carried out directly from the nuclear medicine hot room in special lead containers. The syringes are filled with the radioactive substance by a system of tele-manipulation. The connecting tubes of the needles are then connected to the syringes and they are placed on the plate of a specially devised constant speed automatic injector enveloped in lead. The small connecting tubes between the syringe and the needle also have a special tubular lead covering.

The staff carrying out the operation are duly protected by aprons and lead-bearing rubber gloves. The rise of the contrast material is then checked through a magnifying dial. At the end of the injection, all radioactive material is removed and the small wounds are sutured with catgut stitches.

Two radiograms are then taken for a study of the lymphatic vessels at the root of the thighs, the pelvis and the paraaortic region. After an interval of 24 hours, further radiograms are taken in order to study the adenographic phase in sagittal, lateral and oblique projections respectively. In some cases we resort to all the technical aids that can facilitate and complete the radiographic study, such as direct magnification, tomography, stereography, etc. It has also proved useful to associate radiological examinations with other tests such as urography, retropneumoperitoneum and inferior vena cavography, ultrasound [18, 21, 38, 45, 47, 52]. Follow-up films are usually taken 2—3 weeks after the injection of radioactive contrast material, and then at regular intervals of 2—3 months until the contrast material in the lymph nodes was completely disappeared.

A standard dose of 10 ml of contrast material per foot is administered to each patient. The specific activity of the ^{131}I was at first variable, but recently we have been using materials with a standard activity of 2.5 mCi/ml. Altogether, each patient is given 20 ml of Lipiodol ^{131}I, with a specific activity of 50 mCi. In some cases in which large adenopathies were clinically appreciable we used larger quantities of contrast material (always with an identical specific activity). In other cases, a second injection of contrast material was given in the same quantity at a later date, even soon afterwards.

References

1. Acconcia, A., Fiumicelli, A.: Linfografia degli arti e del piccolo bacino. Radiol. Med. **47**, 461 (1961).
2. Alessandri, R., Biagini, C., Bompiani, C., Fanucci, A., Loasses, A.: La linfoadenografia. Problemi di tecnica e applicazioni alla patologia neoplastica. Radiol. Med. **47**, 458 (1961).
3. — — — — — Presupposti fisiologici e note di tecnica in linfoadenografia. Nuntius Radiol. **27**, 721 (1961).
4. Arnulf, G.: Précisations téchniques sur la lymphographie des membres. Lyon chir. **53**, 772 (1957).
5. — La lymphographie au lipiodol extra-fluide. Lyon chir. **58**, 307 (1962).
6. Arvay, N., Picard, J. D.: L'exploration radiologique des voies lymphatiques. Presse méd. **70**, Suppl. 31, 1962.
7. — — Manlot, G.: Téchnique de la lymphographie abdomino-thoracique. Rev. franç. Étud. clin. biol. **7**, 435 (1962).

8. Asher, W. M., Freimanis, A. K.: Echographic diagnosis of retroperitoneal lymph node enlargement; Ultrasound scanning technique and diagnostic findings. Amer. J. Roentgenol. **105**, 438—445 (1969).
9. Battezzati, M.: La linfografia degli arti: tecnica ed eventuali possibilità diagnostiche. Boll. Soc. Piem. Chir. **29**, 321 (1959).
10. — Contributo della mia Scuola ai problemi di tecnica linfoadenografica. Radiol. Med. **47**, 459 (1961).
11. Baun, S., Bron, K. M., Wexler, L., Abrams, H. L.: Lymphangiography, cavography and urography: comparative accuracy in the diagnostic of pelvic and abdominal metastases. Radiology **81**, 207 (1963).
12. Belanger, R., Maret, C., Onimet-Oliva, D., Katz, L.: Technique de lymphographie par catheter. J. Canad. Radiol. **16**, 237 (1965).
13. Brunn, S., Engeset, A.: Lymphoadenography. A new method for the visualization of the enlarged lymph nodes and lymphatic vessels. Acta Radiol. **45**, 389 (1956).
14. Colin, R.: L'exploration du système lymphatique en pathologie chirurgicale. Acquisitions récentes et résultats pratiques. Presse méd. **68**, 51 (1960).
15. — L'exploration du systéme lymphatique en pathologie chirurgicale. Bordeaux: Union Fran. Impress. Edit., 1961.
16. Collette, J. M.: Lymphographie expérimentale et clinique. Description d'une technique d'opacification radiologique du systéme lymphatique périphérique et du groupe ganglionnaire ilio-pelvien. Acta chir. belg. **54**, 607 (1955).
17. Damascelli, B., Musumeci, R., Uslenghi, C.: Instruments for lymphography. Lymphology **2**, 166 (1969).
18. — Bonadonna, C., Musumeci, R., Uslenghi, C.: Two-dimensional pulsed echo detection of para-aortic lymph nodes. Surg. Gynec. Obstet. **128**, 772—776 (1969).
19. del Buono, M., Fuchs, W. A., Ruttimann, A.: La linfografia: tecnica, indicazioni, diagnostica. Radiologia **15**, 1045 (1959).
20. de Roo, T.: The technique of lymphography. Medicamundi **10**, 101 (1965).
21. — Thomas, P., Kropholler, R. W.: The importance of tomography for interpretation of the lymphographic picture of lymph node metastases. Amer. J. Roentgenol. **94**, 924 (1965).
22. — Eine einfache Technik der Lymphographie. Radiologe **8**, 197—202 (1968).
23. Desprez-Curely, J. P., Bismuth, V., Laugier, A.: Exploration radiologique des lymphonodes ileo-lumbares par lymphographie. Nouv. Rev. franç. Hémat. **2**, 91 (1962).
24. di Matteo, C., Bellucci, M., Morabito, A.: Metodi e tecniche per la linfografia degli arti. Atti Accat. Anat. Chir. **50**, 1 (1959).
25. — Formiconi, E., Bellucci, M., Morabito, A.: La linfoangiografia: modalità, tecniche, risulati e applicazioni cliniche. Progr. Ter. (Milano) **1**, 5 (1961).
26. Dolan, P. A.: The technique of clinical lymphangiography. J. Canad. Ass. Radiol. **15**, 67 (1964).
27. — Moore, E. B.: Improved technique of lymphography. Amer. J. Roentgenol. **88**, 110 (1962).
28. Fischer, H. W.: A technic for radiography of lymph nodes and vessels. Clin. Lab. Invest. **6**, 522 (1957).
29. — Zimmermann, G. R.: Roentgenographic visualization of lymph nodes and lymphatic channels. Amer. J. Roentgenol. **81**, 517 (1959).
30. Gough, M. H., Guiney, E. J., Kinmonth, J. B.: Lymphangiography: new techniques and uses. Brit. med. J. **1963 I**, 1181
31. Kaindl, F., Mannheimer, E., Pfleger-Schwarz, L., Thurnher, B.: Lymphoangiography und Lymphadenographie der Extremitäten. Stuttgart: Thieme 1960.
32. Kenyon, N. M., Soto, M., Viamonte, J. M., Parks, R. E., Farrel, J. J.: Improved techniques and results of lymphography. Surg. Gynec. Obstet. **114**, 677 (1962).
33. Kinmonth, J. B.: Lymphangiography in man. A method of outlining lymphatic trunks at operation. Clin. Sci. **11**, 13 (1952).
34. — Taylor, G. W., Harper, R. K.: Lymphangiography. Technique for its clinical use in lower limbs. Brit. med. J. **1955 I**, 940
35. — Lymphangiography by radiological methods. J. Fac. Radiol. (Lond.) **6**, 217 (1955).

36. KNISK, M., PANNING, W. P.: A simple practical technic of lymphography. Radiology **88**, 576 (1967).
37. KROPHOLLER, R. W., BLOM, J. M. H., IRTO, I.: Lymfografie met behulp van een polytheencatheter. Ned. T. Geneesk. **112**, 696—698 (1968).
38. LEE, B. J., NELSON, J. H., SCHWARZ, G.: Evaluation of lymphangiography, inferior venacavography and intravenous pyelography in the clinical staging and management of Hodgkin's disease and lymphosarcoma. New Engl. J. Med. **271**, 327 (1964).
39. LEENHARDT, P., COLIN, R.: L'exploration lymphatique in vivo. Methodes utilisées, incidents biologiques. Presse méd. **65**, 1534 (1962).
40. LENZI, E., TOTI, A.: Sulla visualizzazione dei linfatici pelvic i con le tecniche linfografiche. Riv. Ostet. Ginec. **16**, 23 (1961).
41. MADDISON, F. E.: Lymphatic cannulation without dye. Radiology **88**, 362 (1967).
42. MALEK, P., BELAN, A., KOLC, J., SUBIN, V.: New technique of demonstrating the superficial as well the deep lymphatic system and its application in clinical practice. IX Int. Congr. Radiol. München 1959.
43. NIIMURA, T.: Intrapelvic lymphadenography. Shinshy Med. J. **7**, 341 (1958).
44. PATTERSON, R. M., RAY, C. T.: Lymphangiography. An improved technique of lymphatic cannulation. Amer. Heart J. **69**, 229 (1965).
45. PUJOL, H., LEMARQUE, J. L.: Ilio-cavographie et lymphographie dans les recherches des adénopathies retropéritonéales. Paris: Masson & Cie 1964.
46. ROSSI, L.: Metodica, valore, limiti e indicazioni dello studio radiologico dell'apparato linfatico mediante linfografia. Atti XXII Congr. Naz. S.I.R.M.—Vol. III, n. 1, 1963.
47. SCHWARZ, G., LEE, B. J., NELSON, J. B.: Lymphography, cavography and urography in the evaluation of malignant lymphomas. (Study of 100 consecutive lymphoma cases.) Acta Radiol. **3**, 138—144 (1965).
48. SEVILLE, M.: La lymphographie. Acta chir. belg. **63**, 678 (1964).
49. THREEFOOT, S. A.: Some chemical, physical and biological characteristics of dyes used to visualise lymphatics. J. appl. Physiol. **15**, 925 (1960).
50. TURNER, A. F.: Lymphangiographic needle clamp. Amer. J. Roentgenol. **96**, 1053 (1966).
51. VIAMONTE, M., JR.: Advances in lymphangiography. Acta Radiol. **2**, 394 (1964).
52. — STEVENS, R. C.: A new trocar for lymphatic cannulation. Radiology **86**, 934 (1966).
53. ZHEUTLIN, N., SHANBROM, E.: Contrast visualisation of lymph nodes. Radiology **71**, 702 (1958).

Chapter 4

Physical Properties of Lipiodol ^{131}I and Dosimetric Studies

GIANNINO FAVA

With 23 Figures

1. Physical-Chemical Properties of Lipiodol Labelled with ^{131}I

Lipiodol is an iodated vegetable oil that has long been used in radiology as a contrast medium in bronchography, myelography, etc. The first research on iodated oils dates back to 1848, but the property of the unsaturated fatty acids of vegetable fats to fix in stable way halogens was discovered only in 1865.

In the preparation of the first iodated oils, it was found that the unsaturated fats fixed an equal quantity of chlorine and iodine and thus produced chloro-iodated oils. Clove oil, however, fixes iodine alone and the resulting compound is called lipiodol. Several types of lipiodol have been prepared with different iodine percentages (by weight). The compounds most frequently used are lipiodol fluid and ultra fluid lipiodol: the former contains 40% by weight of iodine, the latter, 38%.

Lipiodol, like oils in general, has a high viscosity that is increased by the presence of iodine and decreased by a rise in temperature. Lipiodol fluid has a viscosity of 200 cp at 15° C which falls to 60 cp at 40° C; instead the ultra fluid Lipiodol has a viscosity of 52 cp at 15° C which falls to 18 cp at 40° C.

Lipiodol-^{131}I is prepared from lipiodol through a simple exchange reaction, produced by putting lipiodol in contact with ^{131}I in the form of sodium iodide. The reaction itself takes place easily and quickly. In order to obtain 20 ml of lipiodol labelled with 50 mCi of ^{131}I, it is enough to exchange 19 millionths of the stable iodine originally contained in the lipiodol [1].

---

[1] The quantity by weight of 1 mCi of a given radio-isotope can be calculated by the formula:

$$P = \frac{3.7 \times 10^7 \times M}{N \times \lambda} \text{ g/mCi}$$

where M is the mass number
N is Avogadro's number
λ is the decay constant.

In the case of ^{131}I, we have ...

$$P = \frac{3.7 \times 10^7 \times 131}{6.02 \times 10^{23} \times 10^{-6}} = 0.008 \ \mu\text{g/mCi}$$

Therefore, 50 mCi correspond to 40×10^{-8} grams of ^{131}I. On the other hand, 20 ml of lipiodol contains 7.6 grams of iodine. In fact, the ratio between 7.6 and 40×10^{-8} is 19 millionths.

The bond of the iodine with the unsaturated fatty acids of the clove oil is very stable. For this reason, lipiodol does not dissolve easily. It is resistant to boiling and to treatment with concentrated acid solutions, while it is divided by treatment with concentrated alkaline solutions. Lipiodol also has a tendency to loose iodine through the action of heat, and Fig. 4.1 shows the effect of moderate and low temperature on the concentration of iodine.

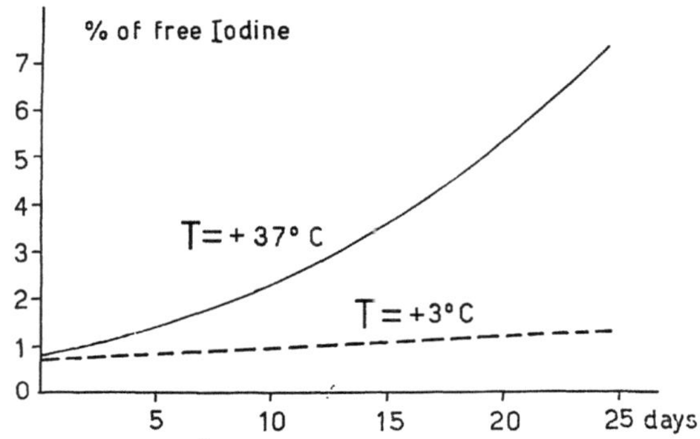

Fig. 4.1. Stability of the iodine bond at low temperature (3° C) and at body temperature. The quantity of free iodine, measured by paper electrophoresis, was negligible at the low temperature and modest at body temperature, 25 days being required for the liberation, in the form of iodide, of 7% of the iodine

The efficiency of the bond between the iodine and the unsaturated fatty acids is shown by the fact that ordinary preparations of Lipiodol-^{131}I contain less than 1% of free iodine. This percentage increases very slowly in time when temperature increases. In order to avoid this disadvantage it is sufficient to keep Lipiodol in a common refrigerator.

Lipiodol is insoluble in water and alcohol, but soluble in ether, gasoline, chloroform, carbon disulphide and fat solvents in general.

Lipiodol, in the form with stable iodine as well as in that with ^{131}I, is used extensively in Europe. In the United States, on the other hand, ethiodol is used. This is ethyl ether of poppy seed oil extraction, containing 37% of iodine by weight. Although there is a great degree of affinity between lipiodol and ethiodol, we would not be entirely justified, biologically speaking, in considering them to be identical in all respects. It is a well-known fact that every living thing has the property of reacting differently in the presence of substances that are chemically related, but not perfectly identical. With this reservation in mind, it is possible to compare, especially from a metabolic point of view, the results obtained from using these two different compounds.

2. Distribution in the Organism

The distribution of lymphatically injected ethiodol-^{131}I has been studied by Seitzman et al. (1963), and in greater detail by Koehler and his collaborators (1964). The values of Seitzman et al. were obtained from measurements on histologic specimens from autoptic material of patients treated by therapeutic lymphangiography.

The results obtained by Koehler et al. are plotted in Fig. 4.2. These results were obtained on fifteen dogs sacrificed on days 3 to 17 after the injection.

An examination of the data reported reveals that about 25% of the activity injected is fixed in the lymphatic system, further 25% to 50% being distributed in the lungs. The remaining 50% to 25% is fairly evenly divided among the other organs, in the main, the liver, kidneys, skin, and bones.

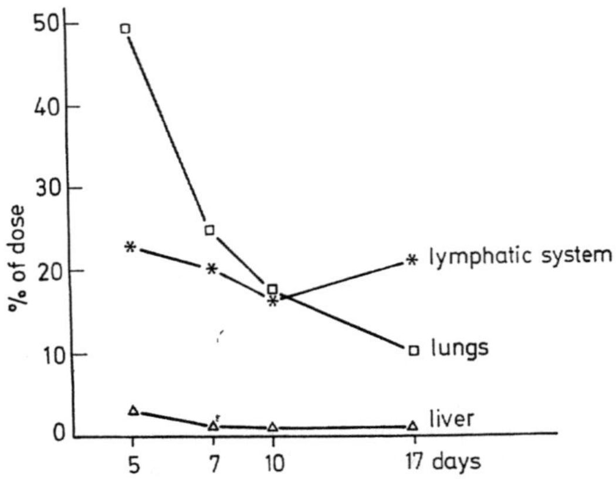

Fig. 4.2. Trend of activity in different tissues after lymphography with Ethiodol-^{131}I. The values are the average obtained from fifteen dogs, studied by Koehler and his collaborators, and sacrificed on days 3 to 17 after the injection

The data of Koehler et al. show that the elimination of radioactivity from the lymphatic system takes place very slowly, while that from the lungs occurs more quickly. This observation leads us to believe that the chemical nature of the radioactive material that accumulates in the lungs is different from that in the lymphatic system and that, furthermore, it consists mainly of free iodine. However, it should also be noted that, according to Seitzman et al. (1963), iodine bound to ethiodol is also found in the lungs.

Fava and Buraggi (1963), and Fava and Roncoroni (1965), have been able to determine the distribution of Lipiodol-^{131}I in man by means of an original external counting technique that will be described further on.

Table 4.1 shows the averaged data from sixty patients who had had Lipiodol-^{131}I injected into the lymphatics of the foot. According to the data reported in the table, an average 22% of the radioactive Lipiodol-^{131}I settled in the lymphatic system and 25% in the lungs.

3. Metabolism

The lymph nodes visualized with lipiodol characteristically retain the contrast medium for a long time, sometimes for as long as a year or more. In 1928, Sicard and Forestier carried out systematic research on the elimination of lipiodol from the body. They concluded that the elimination process is slow but constant, and that the iodine is eliminated in inorganic form mainly in the urine.

Table 4.1. *Values of concentration C of ^{131}I recorded in the lymph nodes and other organs; average values from sixty patients examined. The 25% of Lipiodol-^{131}I which can reach the lung, via the thoracic duct is considerable, although the actual concentration fluctuates between substantially different values. The values of the effective half-lives T_e in various organs demonstrate that, in general, lipiodol is eliminated from the lung much faster than from the lymph nodes. — This exerts considerable influence on the value of the dose which is in direct proportion to T_e itself:*

$$D(\infty)=73.8\,\overline{E}_\beta\, C_0\, T_e \quad \text{rad}$$

$\overline{E}_\beta$: *average energy of the rays emitted by the ^{131}I.*
C_0: *initial concentration of the radioactive substance in the region under consideration.*
T_e: *effective half-life of the radioactive substance in the region under examination.*

Lymph nodes		C µCi/g		T_e days	A_0 as % A. S.	
Inguinal		40.51		9	5.36	
Iliac		39.32		10	9.42	
Lumbar		61.45		7	12.95	
Average values		44.78		9	22.00	
Organ under examination						
Liver		0.0591		4.71	2.10	
Spleen		0.648		4.45	1.24	
Thyroid		3.935		6.54	0.93	
Lung	right	9.4	m 0.5 M 24	5.00	25.00	m 4.3 M 61
	left	8.7	m 0.8 M 20			

A_0 = Maximum activity in a body district at time $t = 0$. A. S. = Total activity administered to the patient. m = minimum. M = Maximum.

It is likely that the iodine is eliminated after it has separated from the lipidic vehicle following the breakdown of the lipiodol molecule by the cells of the tissues with which it comes in contact. The iodine enters in the iodine pool of the body and then follows the fate of the iodine.

With Lipiodol-^{131}I it is possible to carry out detailed research on its own metabolism due to the ease with which the radioactive iodine can be traced. However, it must be noted that all research so far conducted on the metabolism of Lipiodol-^{131}I, hence depending on the radioactivity of the tracer, relates to the metabolism of the iodine and not to that of the lipiodol molecule in toto. Nevertheless, from the radiodiagnostic, as from the radiotherapeutic and dosimetric points of view, iodine is the part of the lipiodol molecule that is of most interest.

a) Elimination from the Body

A practical method for following the elimination of a radionuclide from the body is the "total body count", as used by Bertoli et al. (1968), de Vecchi et al. (1968); they measured the body's total and sectorial radioactivity at regular intervals after the endolymphatic introduction of Lipiodol-^{131}I. With this technique, it is possible to follow the reduction of radioactivity in the body as a result of the decay and elimination of the radionuclide. The half-life of the curve obtained represents the effective half-life (T_e) of the ^{131}I injected into the body with the lipiodol. It is easy to calculate the biological half-life (T_b), i. e. the rate at which the body metabolizes Lipiodol-^{131}I, when the physical half-life (T_p) is known:

Fig. 4.3 shows the radioactivity decay curve for one of the cases studied; it is represented by a single-phase exponential.

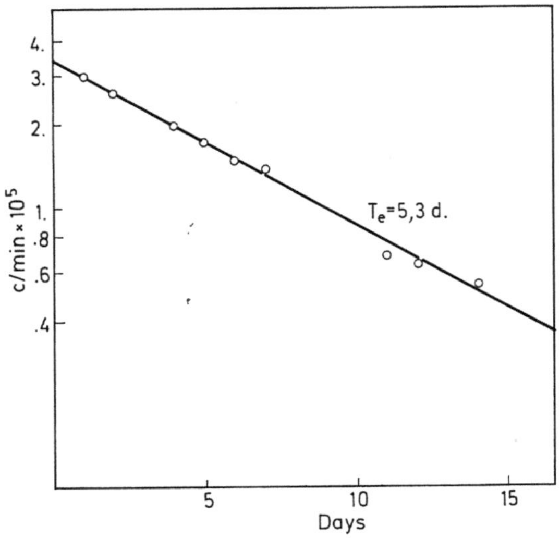

Fig. 4.3. The trend, with the passage of time, of the total activity in the body. The total activity of the body was measured by mechanically moving the scintillator above the patient's body and recording the total number of impulses in correspondence with a body profile survey. As the time used for scanning was known, it was thus possible to express the body activity in terms of counts per minute, a value which was then corrected by subtracting the background radiation. The trend, as indicated on a semi-logarithmic scale, of the data obtained, gives a single-phase exponential curve. The abscissa of the ordinate point equal to ½ of the initial activity supplies the value of the effective half-life: $T_e=5.3$ days

Fig. 4.4 shows a case in which the radioactivity decay curve is represented by a two-phase exponential.

In the case in which the radioactivity decay curve is represented by a two-phase exponential, about 30% of the radionuclide is eliminated at a very rapid rate ($T_e=1.4$ days), while the remaining 70% is eliminated at a normal rhythm ($T_e=7.4$ days). Obviously, the chemical nature of these two fractions is different. No studies have been made to define the two different chemical natures. However, it is probable that the percentage of ^{131}I eliminated at a fast rate is free iodine, or iodine in a state such that it can easily be detached and eliminated. This impression is based on research conducted on the urinary elimination of radioiodine injected as a tracer of the thyroid function (di Pietrantoni, 1967).

Table 4.2 shows the data obtained in some cases studied with the "total body count" technique. The average T_e is approximately 7 days, while the biological T_b is about 60 days. This high value of the biological half-life of the iodine bound to lipiodol explains why the lymph node opacity lasts so long after the endolymphatic injection of lipiodol.

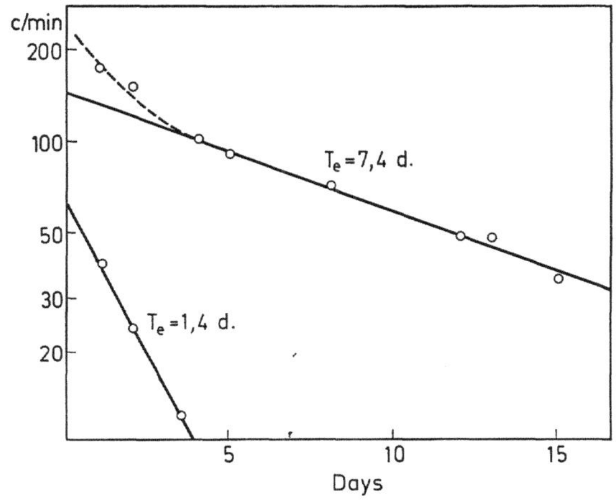

Fig. 4.4. The trend, on a semilogarithmic scale, of a two-phase exponential. The curve reveals after an initial phase of about four days the rapid elimination of 30% of the injected activity (T_e=1.4 days) and a second, decidedly slower, elimination phase (T_e=7.4 days)

Table 4.2. *The trend, with the passage of time, of the total radioactivity of the body following the endolymphatic administration of Lipiodol F-^{131}I, in the more expressive cases*

Case No.	Dose given mCi	T_e days	T_b days	Renovation rhythm %
4	21.4	6.4	31.4	2.20
5	36.2	7.0	53.6	1.29
6	25.4	7.0	53.6	1.29
7	26.8	1.4 (27%)	1.7	40.80
		7.4 (73%)	91.5	0.75
8	44.1	2.7 (37%)	5.0	13.91
		7.2 (63%)	68.2	1.01
9	32.0	5.5	17.3	4.00
10	37.4	5.0	13.2	5.25

b) Elimination

Urine is the main way of eliminating iodine-131 endolymphatically injected as Lipiodol-^{131}I. All the iodine excreted in the urine is in inorganic form (Koehler et al., 1964; Bertoli et al., 1968).

By daily measurements of the activity of iodine-131 present in the urine, expressed as a percentage of the activity injected (corrected for decay), a single-phase exponential curve is obtained, except for the first two or three days, and from this it is possible to calculate the rate at which the iodine is eliminated in the urine (Fig. 4.5).

By comparing this rate with that at which the iodine is eliminated from the body (as calculated from the curves obtained by the "total body count" technique), it is possible to calculate the rate at which the iodine is eliminated in other ways (feces, perspiration, and exhaled air).

Table 4.3 shows the data relative to ten cases, and from this it can be seen that 50—100% of the iodine removed from the body after endolymphography with

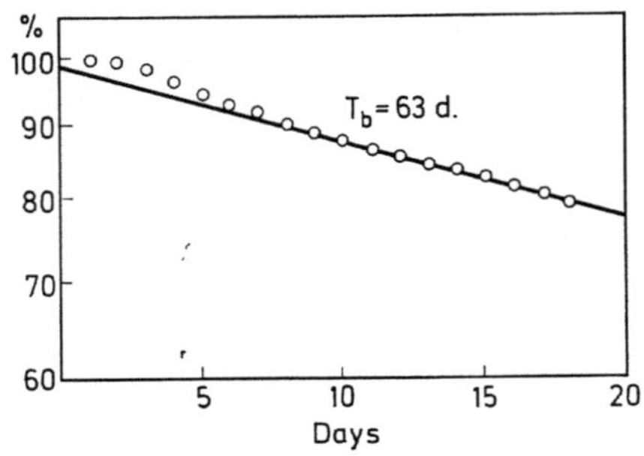

Fig. 4.5. The trend, with the passage of time, of elimination in urine, determined on the basis of daily measurements of the quantity of ^{131}I present in 24-h urine samples over a period of time from 20 to 30 days. Assuming the quantity of Lipiodol F-^{131}I injected to be equal to 100, and subtracting from it the quantity eliminated daily (appropriately corrected for decay), a complete series of values of the residual dose was obtained. These values, when reproduced on a semilogarithmic scale, resulted in a straight line, expressed mathematically by an exponential function. The exponent is the percentage of radioactive substance eliminated, daily, by urinary means (decay rate)

Table 4.3. *Elimination of ^{131}I through urine and other emunctories after endolymphatic administration of Lipiodol F-^{131}I*

Case No.	Renovation rhythm		
	Body R %	Urine R %	Other ways R %
1	—	1.0	—
2	—	3.5	—
3	—	1.3	—
4	2.2	1.6	0.6
5	1.3	1.0	0.3
6	1.1	1.6	0.5
7	2.0 [a]	1.1 [a]	0.9
8	1.03 [b]	1.0	0.03
9	4.0	4.9	—
10	5.3	4.1	1.2

[a] Calculated on 73% of the injected dose.
[b] Calculated on 67% of the injected dose.

Lipiodol-^{131}I is eliminated in the urine. A certain amount of ^{131}I is eliminated through perspiration and (It is well-known that the fecal elimination of iodine ist not important.) the actual amount varies from patient to patient and is conditioned by environmental conditions. The function of perspiration as a vicarious means of excretion, in comparison with that of the urine, is well-known and has also been documented by the research conducted by DI PIETRANTONI (1963) with ^{22}Na.

And lastly, DE VECCHI et al. (1968) have shown that, during the first two days after the lymphatic injection of Lipiodol-^{131}I, there is a slight elimination of ^{131}I through exhaled air (approximately 1‰ of the activity injected). Afterwards, this percentage decreases to a minimum, practically negligible, value.

c) Metabolism in the Blood

The blood lends itself to the study of the metabolism of the tracers contained in it because, unlike the other organs and systems, it can be studied in vitro and the quantity and chemical nature of the tracer contained in it can be very exactly measured. D'AMICO and LUCCHINI (1963) studied the quantity of ^{131}I in the blood by measuring the radioactivity separately, i. e. in organic and inorganic form, as bound to lipidic substances in toto, as well as to non-esterified lipidic substances and to proteins. They obtained a series of curves from which the conclusion can be drawn that about 10% of the iodine present in the blood after lymphography with Lipidol-^{131}I is present in a lipidic molecule.

BERTOLI et al. (1968) have examined the change with the passage of time in the percentage of organic and inorganic iodine in the plasma, as well as that of the iodine bound to the red blood cells, after lymphography with Lipiodol-^{131}I. The values obtained are shown in Fig. 4.6: they are the average of six cases studied. They show that the percentage of iodine in organic form increases from 22% during the first few minutes after injection to 53% after twelve days.

The curve of the activity in the blood (understood as the volume of blood in circulation) expressed in relation to the activity administered and corrected for the

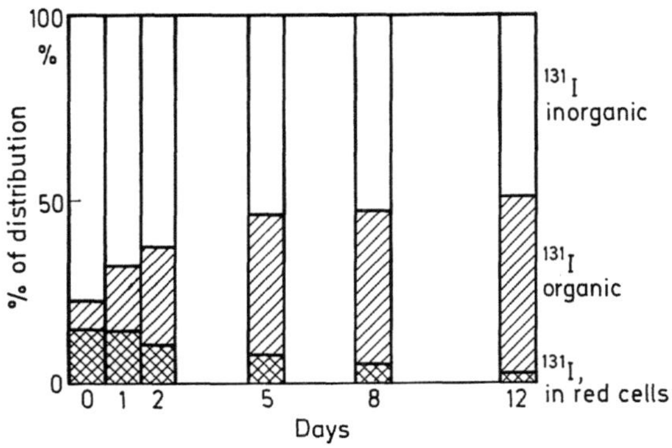

Fig. 4.6. The trend of the percentual distribution of the activity in the different components of the blood (average values obtained from six patients). The percentages of inorganic ^{131}I, and ^{131}I bound to the red blood cells, decrease progressively while the percentage of organic ^{131}I increases considerably

physical decay, shows a progressive increase during the first few days. This is followed by a period of stasis and then by a decrease (Fig. 4.7). This curve shows the trend of the ^{131}I present in the blood as a result of the endolymphatic injection of Lipiodol-^{131}I. The same data can be expressed as a percentage of the residual activity in the body, calculated from the curves described in paragraph 3. a) on the elimination of a radionuclide from the body (Fig. 4.8). The radioiodine in the blood tends to increase relatively to the total iodine present in the body. Thus there is a progressive transfer of radioactivity from the extra-hematic tissues to the blood. Interestingly, this displacement follows a mathematical law represented by a curve, the significance of this being that the activity in the blood tends to a maximum when the time tends to infinity.

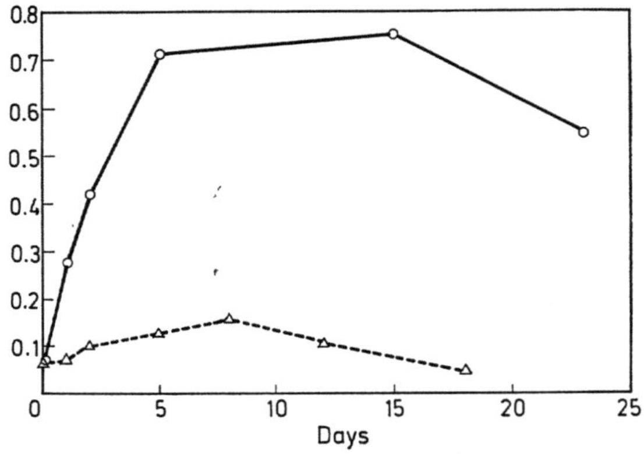

Fig. 4.7. The trend, with the passage of time, of the activity in the blood expressed as a percentage of the dose injected (data corrected for decay). Among the six examined patients we report here the two more expressive cases: it is evident, in both, a progressive increase of the activity in the blood during the first few days, followed by a period of stasis and then by a progressive decrease: ○ patient number 2; △ patient number 3 according to the table III pag. 177 in Bertoli et al.

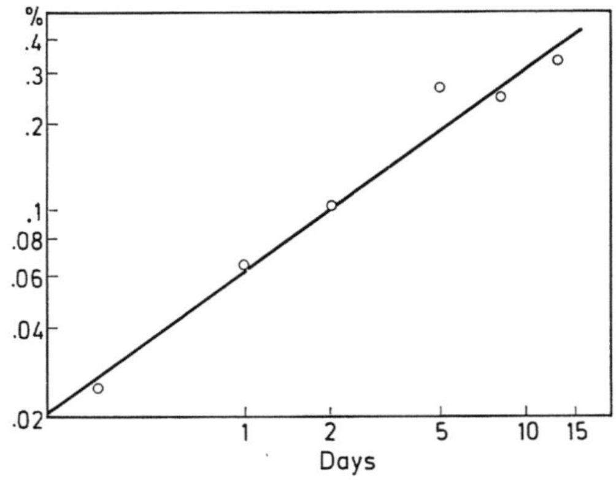

Fig. 4.8. The trend, with the passage of time, of the activity present in the blood expressed as a percentage of the injected dose (values corrected for decay): the equation that mathematically describes this trend will be of the following type: $y=a \cdot x^b$, although obviously within experimental limits. In practice for intervals of time of the order of one month, the activity in the blood increases continuously. After this, the increase becomes somewhat slower and tends to a saturation value

Naturally, this equation is valid only within experimental limits (a month at the very most). However, it has been obtained in all the cases we have studied, even though its parameters assume different values.

d) Metabolism in the Lungs

A substantial fraction of the lipiodol injected reaches the lungs (Section 2) (FAVA, 1966). BAGLIANI et al. (1966) and DE VECCHI et al. (1967) have shown that the radioactivity in the pulmonary area decreases more rapidly than in the abdominal one (Figs. 4.9 a and b).

BERTOLI et al. (1966) have measured at regular intervals the radioactivity present in patients treated with injections of Lipiodol-^{131}I into the lymphatic vessels by recording the so-called "body profile" (Fig. 4.10/Section 5—Paragraph 4). On the body profiles they have measured the area of the part of the curve that corresponded

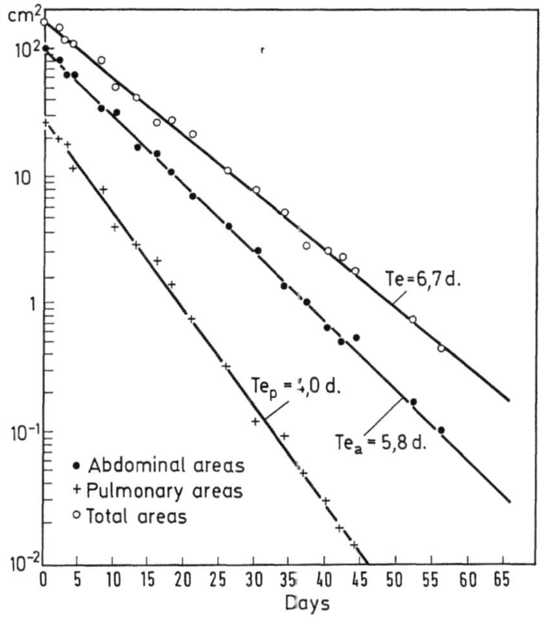

Fig. 4.9 a. The trend, with the passage of time, of the abdominal, pulmonary, and total activity. Values of the activity were obtained from a series of body profiles on all patients up to two months after the lymphography. The areas of the total surface, as well as those of the partial surfaces, subtended from the curve corresponding to the lungs and the abdomen, were then measured with a planimeter on each body profile. These areas were considered to represent, respectively, the average total activity and activity in the pulmonary and abdominal regions. The areas values were then reproduced on a semilogarithmic scale in relation to time. The dates for the different measurements are indicated along the abscissa. A method of this kind makes it possible to express with considerable precision the physical half-lives, insofar as the surface subtended from the body profile indicates the average activity of a region, and thus almost completely eliminates the errors due to the difficulty of repeating the surveys under the selfsame geometric conditions

to the pulmonary, abdominal, and inguinal areas. The ratio between the values of the abdominal and pulmonary areas has shown a constant increase in the cases so far studied (Fig. 4.11).

DE VECCHI et al. (1968) have followed the course of the pulmonary activity with time by measuring the activity exhaled by patients subjected to endolymphatic radiotherapy. This air was filtered for five minutes through 50 grams of activated char-

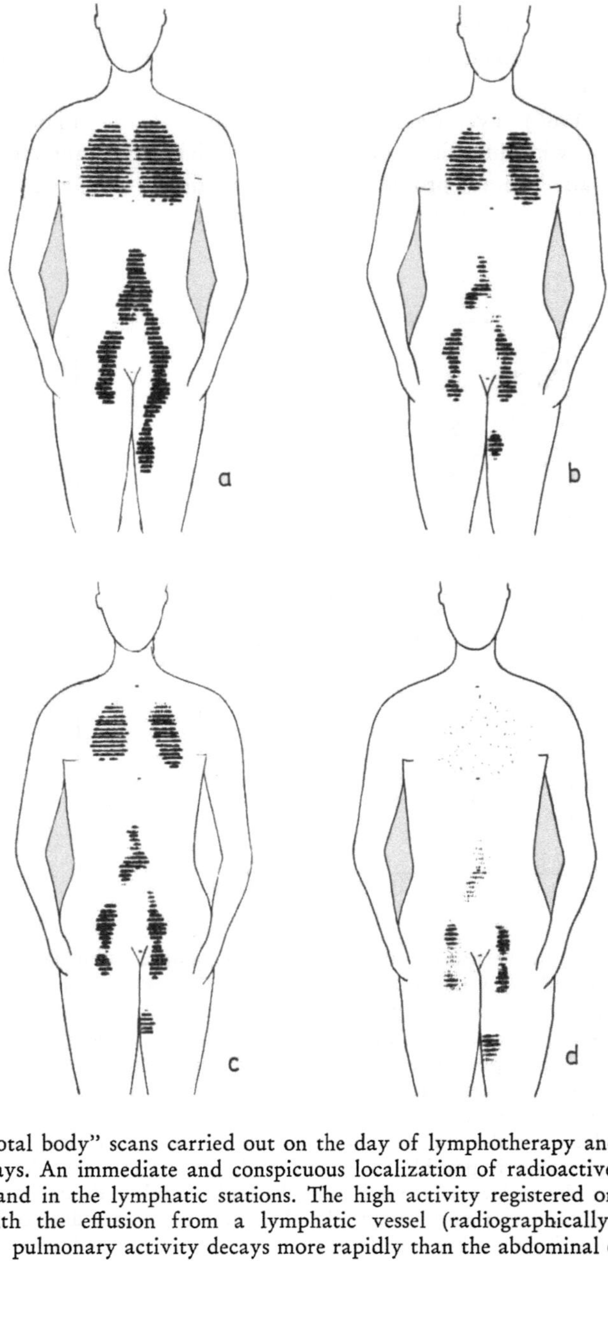

Fig. 4.9 b. "Total body" scans carried out on the day of lymphotherapy and after four, eight and fifteen days. An immediate and conspicuous localization of radioactive material appears in the lungs and in the lymphatic stations. The high activity registered on the left thigh is connected with the effusion from a lymphatic vessel (radiographically confirmed). The pulmonary activity decays more rapidly than the abdominal one

coal. Afterwards, it was subjected to counting. They found that the speed of elimination increases very rapidly during the first one to three hours after the lipiodol has been injected. It then gradually decreases and almost ceases within three to four days.

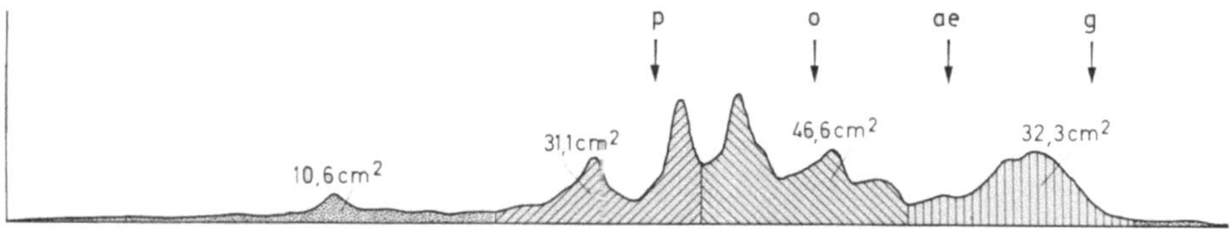

Fig. 4.10. An example of a body profile is here reproduced, complete with the different subdivisions and the corresponding areas subtended from the curve. The small letters indicate the different reference points (*p* = pubis; *o* = navel; *ae* = apophysis; *g* = neck)

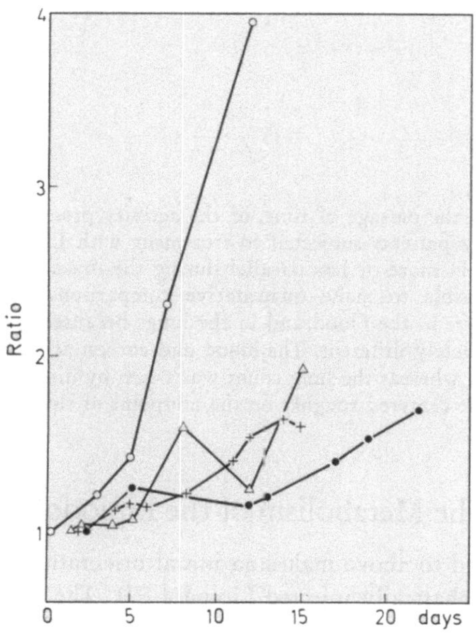

Fig. 4.11. The trend, with the passage of time, of the relationship between abdominal and pulmonary activity as observed in four patients. The initial value was assumed to be 1

A comparison between the trends of the activities in the blood, the lungs, and the exhaled air is interesting. The values, at different times, were recorded on a logarithmic scale. As can be seen from Fig. 4.12, during the initial phase, which lasted from one to two hours (roughly corresponding to the injection of the lipiodol into the feet), the three curves show a more or less identical trend. In particular, a very rapid increase of the activities can be noted in the first few minutes. However, the trends differ considerably in the second phase following the injection of the lipiodol when the patient—once again moving his feet and legs—causes a more rapid movement of the radioactive contrast medium beyond the lymphatic vessels.

The activity in the lungs increases immediately and quickly for a period of twelve to twenty-four hours. In the blood, the activity continues to increase slowly for five or six days while, on the other hand, the activity present in the exhaled air begins to decrease, first rapidly, and then slowly, finally disappearing after three to four days.

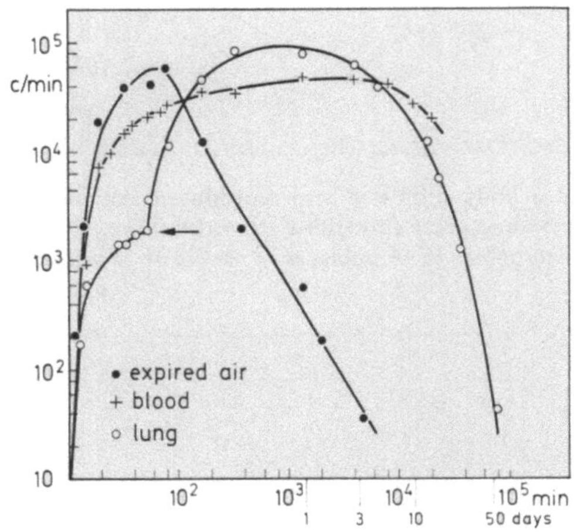

Fig. 4.12. The trend, with the passage of time, of the activity present in the lungs, the blood, and in the air exhaled by patients subjected to treatment with Lipiodol F-^{131}I. One can see how the various trends run more or less parallel during the injection period, but then differ decisively. It is not possible to make quantitative comparisons between the counts/min. recorded in the expired air, in the blood and in the lungs because the geometrical conditions of measurement are completely different. The blood and carbon activity counts were taken in a well counter [NaI(Tl)], whereas the lung count was taken by directional counter [NaI(Tl)] from the outside centered roughly on the midpoint of the right lung field

e) The Metabolism of the Lipiodol-^{131}I

The research referred to above makes an initial orientation possible on the metabolism of the endolymphatically injected Lipiodol-^{131}I. The endolymphatic injection of lipiodol is followed by its distribution in the various tissues, as well as in the lymphatics and the lymph nodes. A significant quantity of lipiodol accumulates in the lungs. The small amounts of free iodine present in the preparation injected are promptly eliminated through the various channels, including the respiratory ones. It is likely that the Lipiodol-^{131}I molecule is broken down by the cells of the tissues in which it has been fixed, and that the ^{131}I enters the "pool" of iodine and follows its metabolism. The breakdown of the Lipiodol-^{131}I molecule occurs more quickly in the lungs so that radioactivity decreases more quickly there than in other organs. In particular, it has been ascertained (DE VECCHI et al., 1968) that the average "T_e" in the lungs is 3.9 days $\pm$ 1.02, while in the abdominal lymph nodes average T_e is 6.3 days $\pm$ 1.24. In the body it has been found that the average T_e is 6.1 days $\pm$ 0.85

An analysis of the results obtained shows that the effective half-life of Lipiodol F-^{131}I in the abdominal lymph nodes is about 1.7 days less than the physical half-life, while in the lungs the elimination of radioactive material occurs more quickly and with the difference that the effective half-life is approximately four days less than that of the physical one.

On the other hand, no lymphatic displacement of radioactive material from the abdominal to the thoracic area has been observed after about the first day after lymphography. Hence the difference between the physical and effective half-life of the ^{131}I in the lymph nodes of the sub-diaphragmatic chain probably reflects a direct and progressive passage of the radioactive material in the form of free iodine, or in a form where it is still bound to the fatty acid molecule, from the individual lymph nodes to the blood, rather than a continuous washing out by the lymph flowing from the feet and legs which, through the thoracic duct, enters the blood stream by passing through the pulmonary cycle.

The shorter effective half-life in the lungs could be due, either to a higher vascularization of the lungs relative to the lymph nodes, or to a particular metabolism of the Lipiodol F-^{131}I in the area of the pulmonary parenchyma. The ^{131}I, on being separated from the Lipiodol, is used partly for the synthesis of thyroxine in the thyroid, and partly eliminated through the urine, perspiration, feces, and exhaled air. Elimination through the urine is the way in which radioactive iodine is usually disposed of, while perspiration is a vicarious means of elimination, although it can assume considerable importance under certain circumstances, and in certain patients. Generally, the biological half-life of the lipiodol iodine is sixty days. This is the reason for the long duration of the opacity of the injected lymph nodes.

4. Counting Techniques

The concentration of ^{131}I-labelled lipiodol in the various parts of the human body can as a rule be determined by the same procedures as those used for any other radioactive substance, viz.,

a) utilizing data derived from studies on animals;

b) utilizing data obtained from counts on autopsy specimens removed from patients treated with labelled lipiodol;

c) by external counting with a specially equipped scintillation counter.

We will now examine this latter procedure in greater detail. As ^{131}I is a γ and β emitter, it is possible to calculate the concentration of the radioisotope (and hence of the labelled lipiodol) by measuring the intensity of the electromagnetic radiation (γ) at the surface of the patient's body. The concentration of radioactivity present in a given sector of the human body can be expressed as the ratio between the actual activity $A(t)$ present, and the weight of the region under examination:

$$C(t) = \frac{A(t)}{\varrho V} \quad \frac{\mu\text{Ci}}{\text{g}}$$

where ϱ is the density of the tissue impregnated with lipiodol, and "V" the volume of the region in question. Once "V" has been determined on the basis of teleradiographies or scan maps, according to appropriate projections of the sector of the human body containing the radioactive source, then the $A(t)$ activity present therein can be deduced by means of a special detector.

As electromagnetic radiation detection is involved, the scintillation counter [NaI(Tl)] is used because of its high efficiency. Moreover, since several contiguous radioactive zones generally appear simultaneously, it is necessary to restrict the detector's visual field. This has to be done in such a way and to such an extent that its response refers, as precisely as possible to the region of interest. For this purpose, detector's sensitive part [which is made of NaI(Tl) crystal] is surrounded by a shield (collimator). This shield, or collimator, is designed in such a way that only the γ radiation from the sector to be explored reaches the crystal itself (Fig. 4.13).

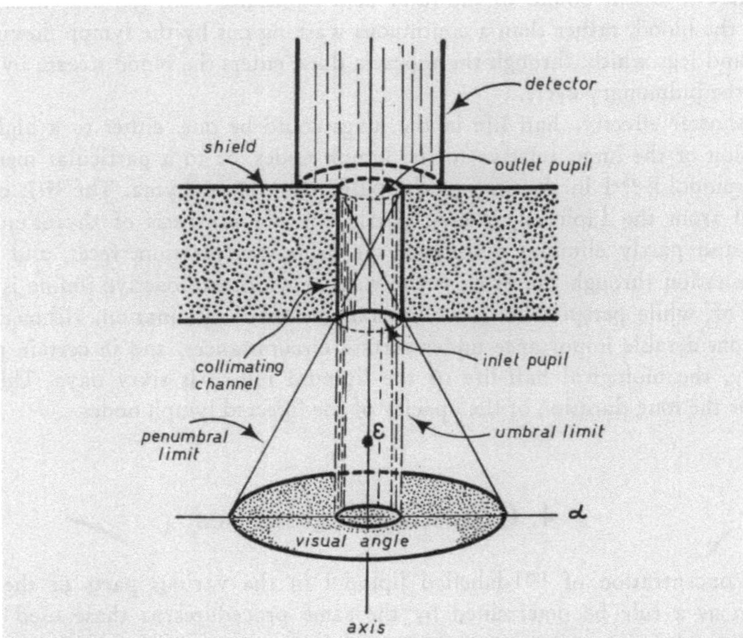

Fig. 4.13. Drawing of a collimator and its relative visual field. The collimator's outlet pupil (internal pupil) defines the area of the crystal detector's sensitive surface, while the inlet pupil (external pupil) and the optical channel determine the form and geometric limits of the detector's visual field. Consequently, two areas can be distinguished in the visual field: the "umbra" or complete shadow, and the "penumbra" or partial shadow. The "umbra" area is the region from which the rays can reach the collimated detector's sensitive surface without encountering any obstacle whatsoever; the "penumbra" is the region from which only some of the rays can reach the collimated detector's sensitive surface, as the remaining area is blocked by components of the collimator itself

As the radiation detected is electromagnetic, the most efficacious shielding material is Pb and the collimation system constitutes the end portion of the probe or, in other words, the unit itself: the photo multiplying tube + the crystal + the collimator. Under these conditions, the amplitude of the detector's visual field clearly depends on the geometric characteristics of the collimator's optical channel. Thus, one has a cylindrical collimator when the optical channel is an upright cylinder coaxial with the probe; a conical collimator when the optical channel is an upright truncated cone coaxial with the probe; a slotted collimator when the optical channel is a rectangular-base truncated pyramid, etc.

Therefore, we need to know exactly how the crystal "sees" through the collimator. In other words, it is essential to know the shape and dimensions of the visual field. The probe's response to the activity of a given source, for a given collimator, will depend on the position occupied by the source within the visual angle. More precisely speaking, by systematically shifting the source, one finds that there are points within the visual field for which the detecting system always gives the same response. All these points taken together form a set of surfaces (isoresponse surfaces); as these are symmetrical in respect to the axis of the probe, we in practice consider the intersection lines that they form with a plane passing through the axis of the probe.

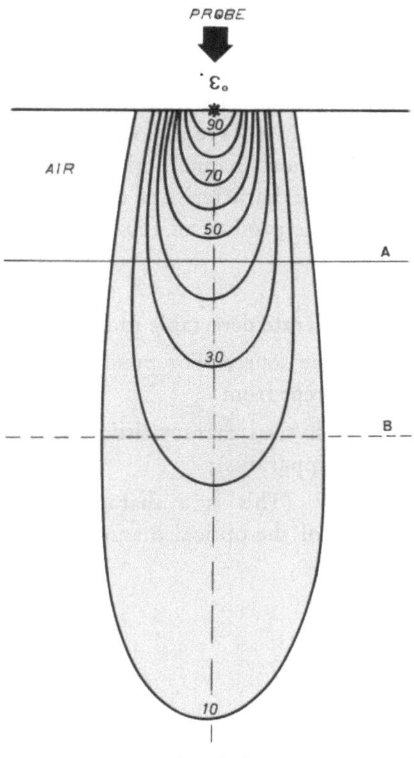

Fig. 4.14 a. An example of the progression of a family of isoresponse curves on the plane containing the probe's axis

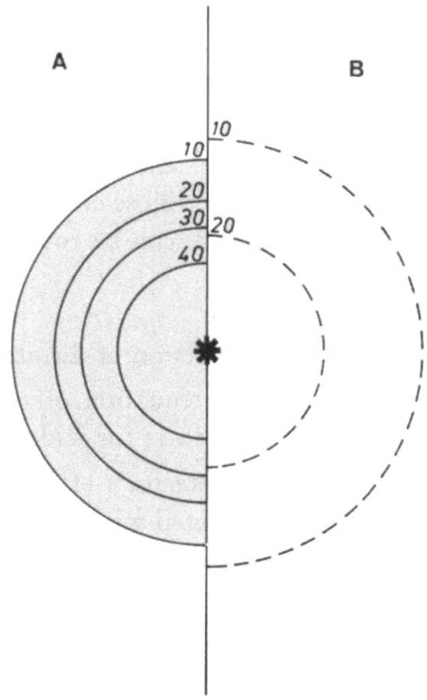

Fig. 4.14 b. For the same source as illustrated in Fig. 14 a, here are shown the sections of the isoresponse surfaces on two planes (*A* and *B*) perpendicular to the probe's axis. The progression of these curves clearly shows the symmetrical character of the isoresponse surfaces in respect to the probe's symmetry axis

In this way, sets of "isoresponse curves" are obtained, the shape of which, for a given collimator, depends on various factors: for instance, on the quantic energy of the radiation emitted by the radionuclide used; on the shape and dimensions of the radioactive source; on the quality and extent of the diffusion medium containing the source itself, etc.

It would obviously be very complex to anticipate the shape of these curves from a purely mathematical point of view. For this reason, therefore, it is generally preferable to establish them experimentally by systematically moving a standard source within a patient-simulating phantom, so as to reproduce each time, in the most precise and realistic way possible, the actual conditions that can arise in various clinical cases (Figs. 4.14 a and b). Once the isoresponse curves (which are characteristic of the collimator being used) have been obtained, it will be possible to determine the radioactive concentration within a given region by following different procedures according to each case. The activity present in the radioactive source can, in fact, be expressed as the ratio between the net counts registered per minute over the localization and the total efficiency of the detector:

$$A(t) = \frac{C\,P\,M\,(t) - C'\,P'\,M'\,(t)}{\varepsilon_0}\ \mu\text{Ci}$$

where: $C\,P\,M\,(t)$ = number of counts registered per minute in relation to the localization,

$C'\,P'\,M'\,(t)$ = background,

ε_0 = total efficiency. A collimated detector's total efficiency depends on numerous factors. Some of them have a close connection with the geometric form of the optical channel, while others have a close connection with the source characteristics, etc.

Total efficiency can be roughly expressed as the product of four factors,

$$\varepsilon_0 = f\,\eta\,s\,g$$

where: f = the fraction of disintegrations that generate detectable radiations;

η = the attenuation of the radiation in the source. For point sources, this is equal to 1; for wide sources, it is different from 1;

s = the detector's efficiency. (This is a physical characteristic that is strictly connected with the electronics of the apparatus);

g = the collimator's geometric efficiency. (This is a characteristic that is closely connected with the geometry of the optical channel and the position of the source in the visual angle);

$$g = \frac{A}{4\pi\,(a+x)^2}$$

where: a = the length of the optical channel,

x = the distance of the source from the plane of the inlet pupil,

A = the area of intersection between the surface of the inlet pupil of the collimator projected from the source point "P", and the sensitive surface of the detector (Fig. 4.15).

Because of the ε_0 expression, it would be complicated to determine its value theoretically, consequently, it is preferable to determine it experimentally. In practice, as far as ε_0 is concerned, one takes the response of the entire detecting system (as expressed in counts per minute) *to the activity of a point source, equal to 1 μCi, placed on the axis of the probe at a distance from the inlet pupil, equal to the length of the optical channel of the collimator.*

Therefore, ε_0 makes it possible to express every measurement recorded directly in the unit of activity.

Let us now suppose that we wish to determine the concentration of radioactivity in the thyroid. This is an example of a small source (the thyroid) in a limited scattering medium (the neck).

The collimator generally used for these measurements is of the type with a cone-shaped optical channel. Therefore, the isoresponse curves to be subsequently taken into consideration will be those obtained with a conical collimator for a small-sized source within a limited scattering medium.

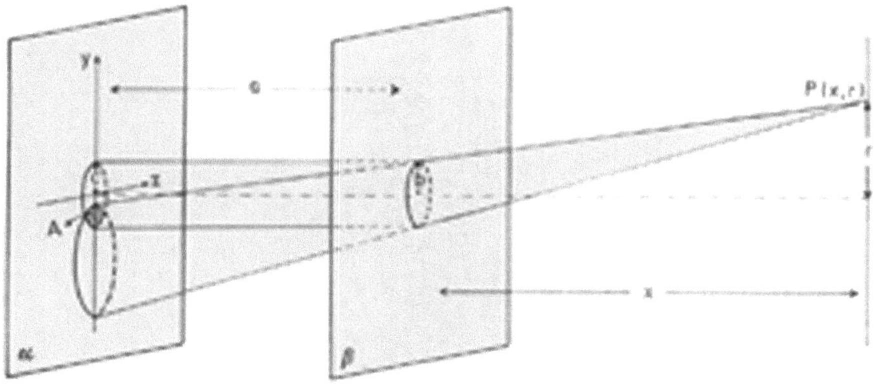

Fig. 4.15. By the geometric efficiency of a collimated detector we mean the ratio between the number of particles that strike the detector's sensitive surface (as limited by the shape of the internal pupil) and the actual number of particles emitted by the source. This ratio can be expressed in relation to the geometric magnitudes that characterize the collimator itself, i. e.,

$$g = \frac{A}{4\pi (a+x)^2}$$

where: a = the length of the collimator's optical channel,
x = the distance of the source from the plane of the collimator's external pupil,
A = the intersection between the surface of the collimator's external pupil projected from the source point P, with the sensitive surface of the detector.

Also shown in the diagram are:
α: the plane of the detector,
β: the plane of the external pupil of the collimator,
b, c: the radii of the collimator's external and internal pupils respectively (for a cylindrical type collimator, $b=c$).

The schematic picture of the source (in this case, the thyroid gland) is superimposed on the set of isoresponse curves in such a way as to coincide with its real position in the collimator's visual angle (Fig. 4.16).

The concentration (assuming that the radioactive substance is uniformly distributed throughout the organ) can be calculated with the formula:

$$C(t) = \frac{C\,P\,M(t) - C'\,P'\,M'(t)}{\varepsilon_0\, \varrho \sum_1^n V_i\, K_i}\ \frac{\mu\text{Ci}}{\text{g}}$$

where: the net counts per minute recorded appear in the numerator,

ε_0 = total efficiency, defined beforehand,

ϱ = density of the impregnated tissue,

V_i = portions of the gland contained between two contiguous isoresponse curves,

K_i = a factor that takes into consideration the proportion to which the quantity of radioactive substance, present in the volume "V_i", contributes to the recorded activity.

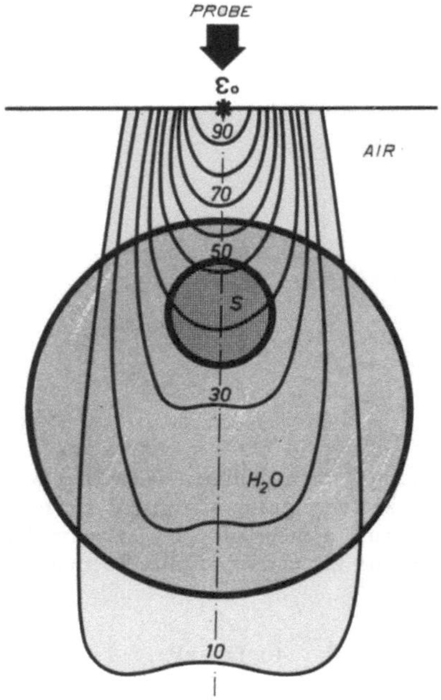

Fig. 4.16. How the isoresponse curves are used to determine the concentration of the radioactivity in the thyroid. The standard curves, plotted for a limited sample-source in a limited diffusion medium, are superimposed on a schematic representation of the organ under examination. As can be seen, the source is contained between the 30% and 60% isodose curves. As a result, it is divided in three sectors in which K_i varies, ordinately, between 0.58 and 0.50; between 0.50 and 0.40; and between 0.40 and 0.35. The various portions of the source volume V_i contained between two contiguous isoresponse curves are evaluated here by thinking of them as composed of many parts, each of which is assimilable with a solid volume calculable in an elementary way. (For similar procedures applied to liver and lungs, see Figs. 4.19 and 4.20)

Fig. 4.16 shows how, in the case being examined, the source is entirely contained between the 60% and the 30% curves. It can thus be divided into three parts in which K varies between 0.58 and 0.50; 0.50 and 0.40; and 0.40 and 0.35.

Another case that can occur is that of a small source in an unlimited scattering medium. This is precisely the situation one is confronted with when one has to consider a thoracic or an abdominal localization, for example, when one wants to determine the concentration of radioactivity within a single lymph node. The situation here is very complex, as it is not possible to locate one node at a time. On the contrary, one is dealing with a group of sources that will influence the crystal of the probe in different ways, not only on account of their different positions in space, but also because they will have absorbed different amounts of the radioisotope [2].

Instead of considering each lymph node separately within the region under examination and then determining the activity in relation to its position in the measuring angle, one considers rather the set of lymph nodes as a whole, as seen by the probe, and then calculates the average C_0 concentration. In this case, too, a cone-shaped optical channel collimator is usually used. By superimposing the iso-

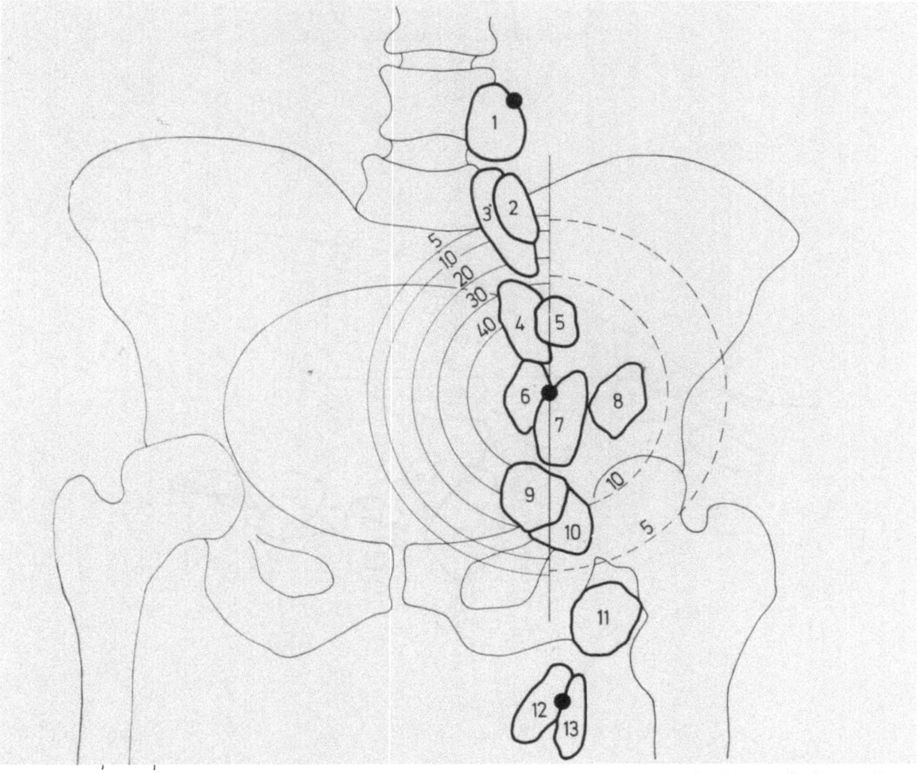

Fig. 4.17. The distribution diagram of the lymph nodes on the coronal plane of the patient is obtained from the teleradiograph of the patient's abdomen in antero-posterior projection. The depth factor f_i can be determined by superimposing on the radiograph the family of isodose curves on the probe's two coronal planes, *a* and *b*, which limit the distribution of the lymph nodes in the measuring angle, and by taking into account the deductions which can be made from Fig. 4.18

response curves determined according to the probe's coronal and sagittal plane on the teleradiographs taken from latero-lateral and antero-posterior positions, respectively, it is possible to locate the lymph nodes fairly accurately within the measuring angle and at the same time to establish the "depth factor" "f_i" for each of them.

---

[2] The adjective "limited" here refers to a volume that is completely contained within the collimator's visual angle. An *unlimited* volume includes the visual angle in its entirety.

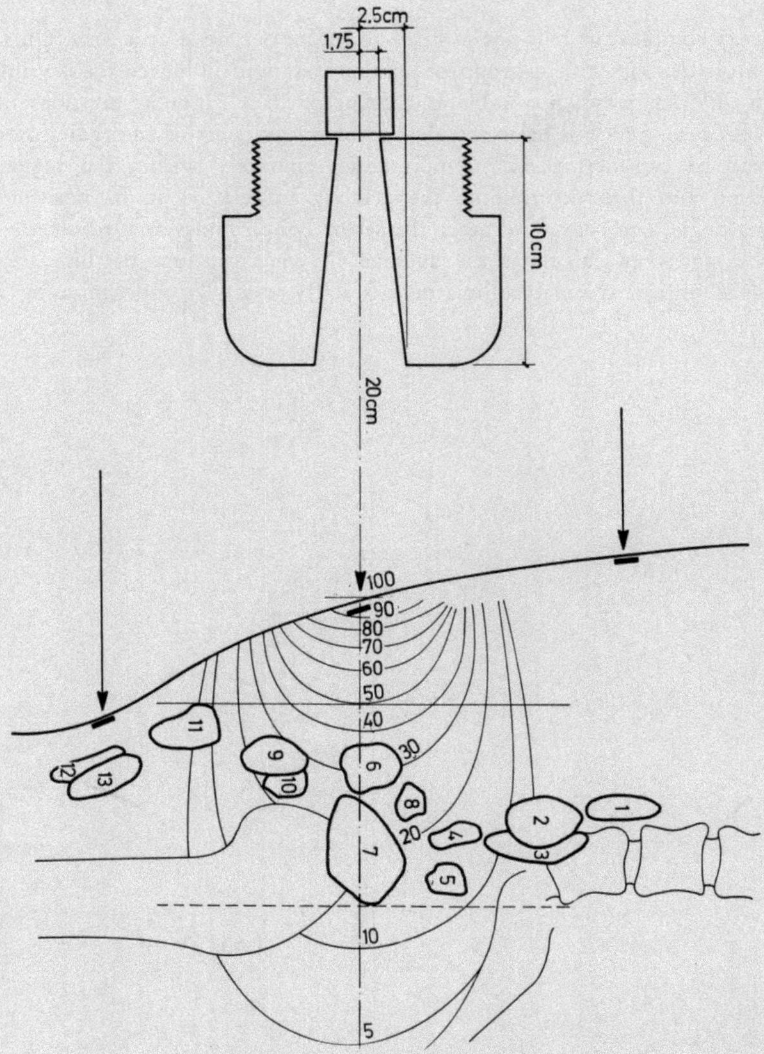

Fig. 4.18. The distribution diagram of the lymph nodes, on a plane passing through the probe's axis and parallel to the sagittal plane of the patient, can be obtained from the teleradiograph of the patient's abdomen in latero-lateral projection. The family of isodose curves on the sagittal plane of the probe is then superimposed on this radiograph. From the diagram thus obtained, the "depth factor" f_i can be calculated for each lymph node included in the measuring angle (also taking into consideration the deductions from Fig. 4.17). The lines *a* and *b* mark the intersections of the system with the two planes that limit, in depth, the distribution of the lymph nodes themselves. Once the "depth factor" f_i for each lymph node is known, the total activity included in the measuring angle is given by:

$$A(t) = f_2 V_2 C(t) + f_3 V_3 C(t) + \ldots + f_{11} V_{11} C(t) \ \mu\text{Ci}$$

considering "$C(t)$" as being constant

$$A(t) = C(t)\,(f_2 V_2 + f_3 V_3 + \ldots + f_{11} V_{11}) \ \mu\text{Ci}$$

where V_i is determined in an elementary way by assuming each lymph node to be either a sphere or an ellipsoid

The factor f_i states in which proportion the radioactivity present in i-th lymph node, situated at a certain point in the measuring angle, contributes to the recorded activity (Figs. 4.17 and 4.18).

Lastly, the various "V_i" volumes of the lymph nodes are calculated by assuming that they are, according to each individual case, either an ellipsoid, or a sphere. (The length of the radius of the sphere or the semi-axis of the ellipsoid, is established by studying two teleradiographs, one taken from a latero-lateral position, and the other from an antero-posterior position, of the lymphatic region being examined.) Therefore, on the basis of what has so far been stated, the average concentration of lipiodol present in a lymph-node region can be expressed as follows:

$$C(t) = \frac{CPM(t) - C'P'M'(t)}{\varrho\, \varepsilon_0 \sum_{1}^{n} i\, f_i V_i} \frac{\mu\text{Ci}}{\text{g}}$$

n = the number of lymph nodes present in the region under examination,
ε_0 = the total efficiency,
ϱ = the density.

When one wishes to determine the concentration of radioactivity in an extensive source, such as the liver or the spleen, it is not the localization of the source in the measuring angle which is important, but the mass of the organ in the solid angle under which the crystal "sees" through the collimator.

Hence, on focusing the probe, this time equipped with a cylindrical optical channel type collimator, on the particular organ of the patient which we wish to examine, and assuming that the radioisotope is uniformly distributed, then the actual concentration is given by:

$$C(t) = \frac{CPM(t) - C'P'M'(t)}{\varepsilon_0\, \varrho \sum_{1}^{n} i\, V_i K_i} \frac{\mu\text{Ci}}{\text{g}}$$

where: ε_0 is always equal to the total efficiency and ϱ is the density, but where V_i now indicates the rotational volume included between two successive isoresponse curves and K_i is a factor which, like the "depth factor" cited in the case of the lymph nodes, takes into account the proportion according to which the radioactivity present in the volume "V_i" contributes to the total recorded activity (Fig. 4.19). These factors, K_i and V_i, can be determined by superimposing the isoresponse curves, obtained for the case of an unlimited source in an unlimited scattering medium, on the transverse axial tomographs of the region being examined which have themselves been recorded in relation to the point of intersection of the axis of the probe with the patient's skin.

Calculating the concentration of radioactivity in the lungs again involves a case of an unlimited source. But this time, the $C(t)$ determination is an extremely complex problem, because the volume and consequently density of the organ involved are not constant.

On the assumption that the activity contained in the lungs does not vary appreciably during the measuring time, then it naturally follows that $C(t)$ varies with the passage of time.

To be more precise: assuming that, with the passage of time, the pulmonary volume oscillates between a minimum (the volume at the end of an exhalation) and a maximum (the volume at the end of an inhalation) [3], then it can be presumed that the $C(t)$ concentration can be described by a harmonic type function:

$$C(t) = \frac{C_1 + C_2}{2} + \frac{C_2 - C_1}{2} \sin\left(\frac{2\pi}{T_v} t + \varphi\right)$$

where: C_1 = the value of the minimum concentration.
C_2 = the value of the maximum concentration.
T_v = the ventilation period (which can generally be assumed to last about 4 seconds).

At this point, another factor that complicates the problem of determining $C(t)$ has to be taken into consideration. As a consequence of the variation in volume

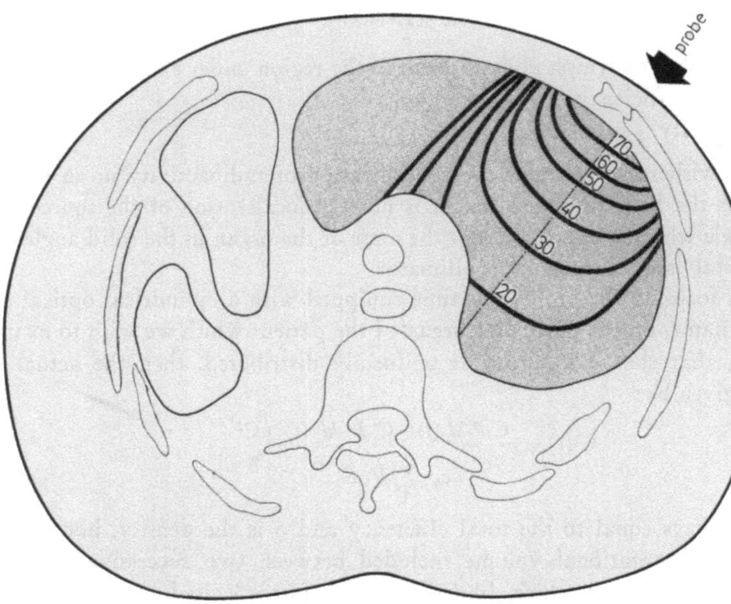

Fig. 4.19. Method of measuring hepatic activity. The family of isoresponse curves is superimposed on the transverse, axial tomograph of the area being examined. The tomograph was effected at the height of the intersection point of the probe's axis with the patient's skin. The curves that define the real limits of the visual field are all contained within the source itself. The plotted diagram makes it possible to determine with a sufficient degree of accuracy which portion of the hepatic mass actually contributes to the count, as well as the variability interval of Ki. The liver occupies all the area between the 10% and the 80% curves; as a consequence, K_i varies theoretically with a continuity between 0.10 and 0.80. In practice, as regards the efficiency of each zone being examined, the average value of the two curves is assumed

that occurs during a measurement effected on the patient, the distance between the source and the probe will vary in time. As a result of this fact, even the ε_0 efficiency (depending essentially on the distance between the probe and the patient's skin) will

[3] We refer to normal, unforced breathing.

oscillate between two values corresponding to the minimum and maximum distances between the source and the surface of the patient's chest. If we wish to calculate $C(t)$ as accurately as possible, we must consider two sets of isoresponse curves, i. e. one recorded for a phantom-probe distance equal to the distance probe to chest surface at the end of a normal inhalation (maximum volume of the source), and the other for a distance equal to the distance probe to chest at the end of a normal exhalation (minimum volume of the source).

The two efficiency values ε_{01} and ε_{02} are recorded in these two extreme situations. We then superimpose the sets of curves for minimum and maximum distance on transverse axial tomographs of the lungs taken under conditions of maximum and minimum volume, respectively. It will then be possible to determine the V_i volumes included in both cases between the two continuous isoresponse curves (Fig. 4.20).

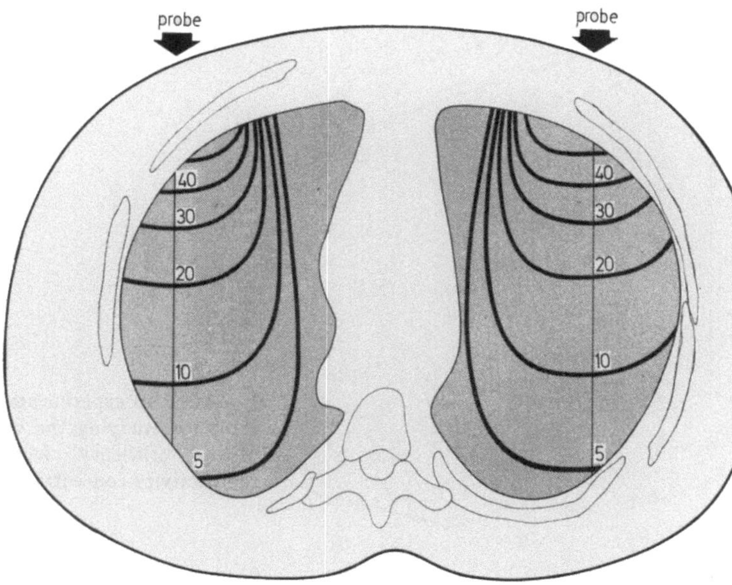

Fig. 4.20. Theoretical method of measuring pulmonary activity. The procedure for measuring hepatic activity is also applicable here. In practice, it is impossible to determine experimentally, as for the liver, the isoresponse curves for an "unlimited" lung simulating standard source. Consequently, the problem of calculating the dose given to the lung is resolved by means of a simple "efficiency" measurement, i. e. when the response of the entire measuring system is known for an activity source that is similar to the lung, and under ambient conditions and in circumstances analogous to those that are present when the patient is operated on, then the activity present in the lung can be determined by the relation:

$$A(t) = \frac{CPM(t)}{\varepsilon}\ \mu\text{Ci}$$

where: "$A(t)$" = the activity that one wishes to know.
"$CPM(t)$" = the net count recorded per minute in connection with the patient's lung.
ε = the efficiency, here, is the response (in net counts per minute) of the entire counting system to the activity of 1 μCi present in the lung-simulating source

Ultimately, the $C\,(t)$ concentration can be expressed as follows:

$$C\,(t) = \frac{C\,P\,M\,(t) - C'\,P'\,M'\,(t)}{\frac{\varepsilon_{01}+\varepsilon_{02}}{2} \cdot \frac{\varrho_1+\varrho_2}{2} \sum_1^n i \, \frac{V_{1i}+V_{2i}}{2} \, K_i} \; \frac{\mu\text{Ci}}{\text{g}}$$

where average values have been considered for all the quantities that vary with the passage of time.

The variation of the "efficiency" factor with varying concentration was demonstrated by means of a few simple measurements made with a paraffin phantom in which 25 small capsules had been placed in a regular pattern, as shown according in Fig. 4.21. Each capsule contained 10 μCi of ^{131}I to give a total activity of 250 μCi. Assuming the distribution to be continuous, varying the distance between the capsules is the same thing as varying the radioactive concentration. The dependence of the efficiency ε_0 upon C is clear enough: for instance, for a 30.57% C variation (between "V" = 1,500 cc. and "V" = 2,160 cc.), there is a 43.23% variation of ε_0.

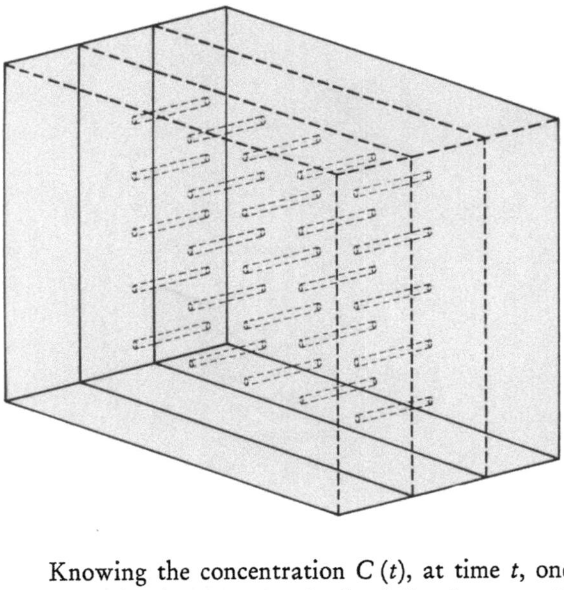

Fig. 4.21. An experimental apparatus for studying the variation of the "efficiency" factor with radioactivity concentration

Knowing the concentration $C\,(t)$, at time t, one can calculate the initial concentration value by reasoning in the following way. In general, the period required for the absorption of lipiodol by the tissues of the various organs is short (a few hours) in comparison with the elimination time. Hence, the absorption time may be disregarded, and the dose absorbed by the tissues because of the presence of the radioactive substance in them is considered as essentially correlated with the elimination period.

Thus, one assumes that absorption is practically instantaneous, after which, within the limits of experimental approximation, radioactive concentration decreases according to the exponential law.

The elimination of the radioactive substance from the tissues is characterized by a "biological half-life", expressed by the formula $T_b = \frac{\ln 2}{\lambda_b}$ sec (where λ_b is the fractional decrease of radioactivity in the tissues per unit of time due exclusively to biological factors). One may therefore conclude that the effective half-life can be expressed by $\frac{1}{T_e} = \frac{1}{T_p} + \frac{1}{T_b}$ sec^{-1}, where T_b is the quantity defined above, and T_p is the "physical half-life" characteristic of the radioisotopes used and depending on the "physical decay constant" λ_p (atom fractions that decay in the time unit), as obtained by the formula:

$$T_p = \frac{\ln 2}{\lambda_p} \text{ sec.}$$

While T_p is characteristic of the radioisotope used, T_b depends strictly on the organ under examination. For this reason, T_e will have different values for different regions. These values can be found experimentally by plotting on a graph having as its ordinate (on a logarithmic scale) the values of the activities measured at different time intervals, and as the abscissa (on a normal scale) the time values corresponding to the different measurements. Within the limits of the approximation made on the assumption that the concentration (or the activity) has an exponential law, this graph will be a straight line.

By extrapolating this straight line to zero, it will be possible to determine the value of the initial concentration $C(o)$ which, in turn, depends on $C(t)$, the concentration at time t from the exponential formula:

$$C(o) = C(t)\, \epsilon^{-\frac{0.693}{\mathrm{Te}} \cdot t} \frac{\mu\mathrm{Ci}}{\mathrm{g}}$$

and the T_e value, as the abscissa of the point which has an ordinate value of $\frac{C(o)}{2}$.
[The reasoning involved can be made, in its entirety, by also referring directly to the measured activity $A(t)$.]

5. Linear Scanning

In "body profile" linear scanning, a detector equipped with a slot-type collimator (a slot placed perpendicular to the direction of movement of the detector) explores the organism by moving along a predetermined axis which may be either parallel or normal to the longitudinal axis of the body (Fig. 4.22).

As the collimator has a truncated-pyramid type optical channel, the detector analyzes the patient according to sections normal to the sagittal plane of the patient. The signals emitted by the detecting probe reach the rate-meter unit which has a linear recording stylus connected to its outlet.

Since the paper unwinds under the point of the stylus in perfect synchronism with the movement of the probe, a continuous "body profile" line is obtained.

The points of this continuous "body profile" will have, as abscissa, the interaction of the transverse section be examined with the sagittal plane of the patient and, as ordinate, the activity included in the section.

The profile thus obtained gives a quantitative indication of the distribution of the radioactive substance throughout the patient's body. The total area covered by the profile, as well as the total count (both done immediately after the introduction of the radioactive lipiodol), can be considered a significant expression of the mCi of ^{131}I injected into a patient receiving endolymphatic therapy.

Thus, the body profiles supply a comprehensive picture of the radioactivity in the organism, making possible an orientative evaluation of its distribution; furthermore, when successive scans are done, it becomes possible to establish the rate at which the total activity decreases, as well as that of the activity in various regions (Fig. 4.23).

In point of fact, by comparing the successive body profiles with the first one, one can find the effective period ("T_e") of the ^{131}I throughout the entire body and, if partial areas are compared, the effective period in the various sectors (Fig. 4.10).

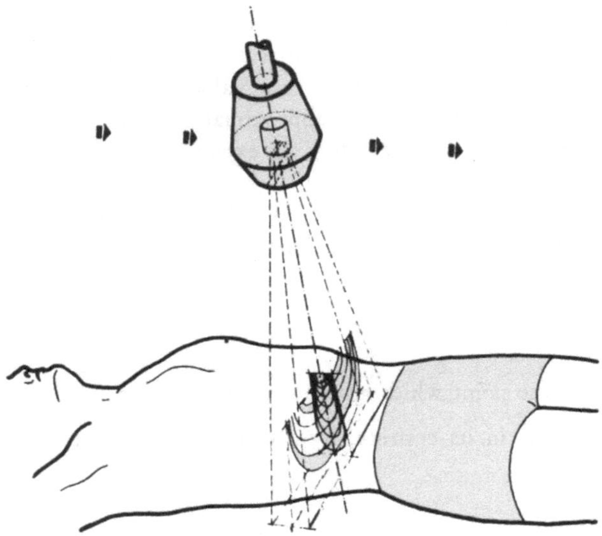

Fig. 4.22. Drawing representing the geometric situation during the recording of a body profile

6. Dosimetry

Knowing the initial concentration and the effective half-life, as obtained from the elimination curve, it is possible to calculate the dose absorbed by the tissues due to the contribution of the β particles and the γ radiations. Since the ^{131}I is a β and γ emitter according to the decay spectrum,

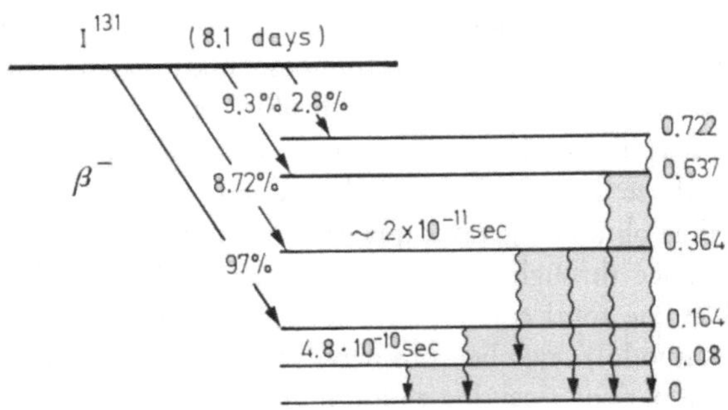

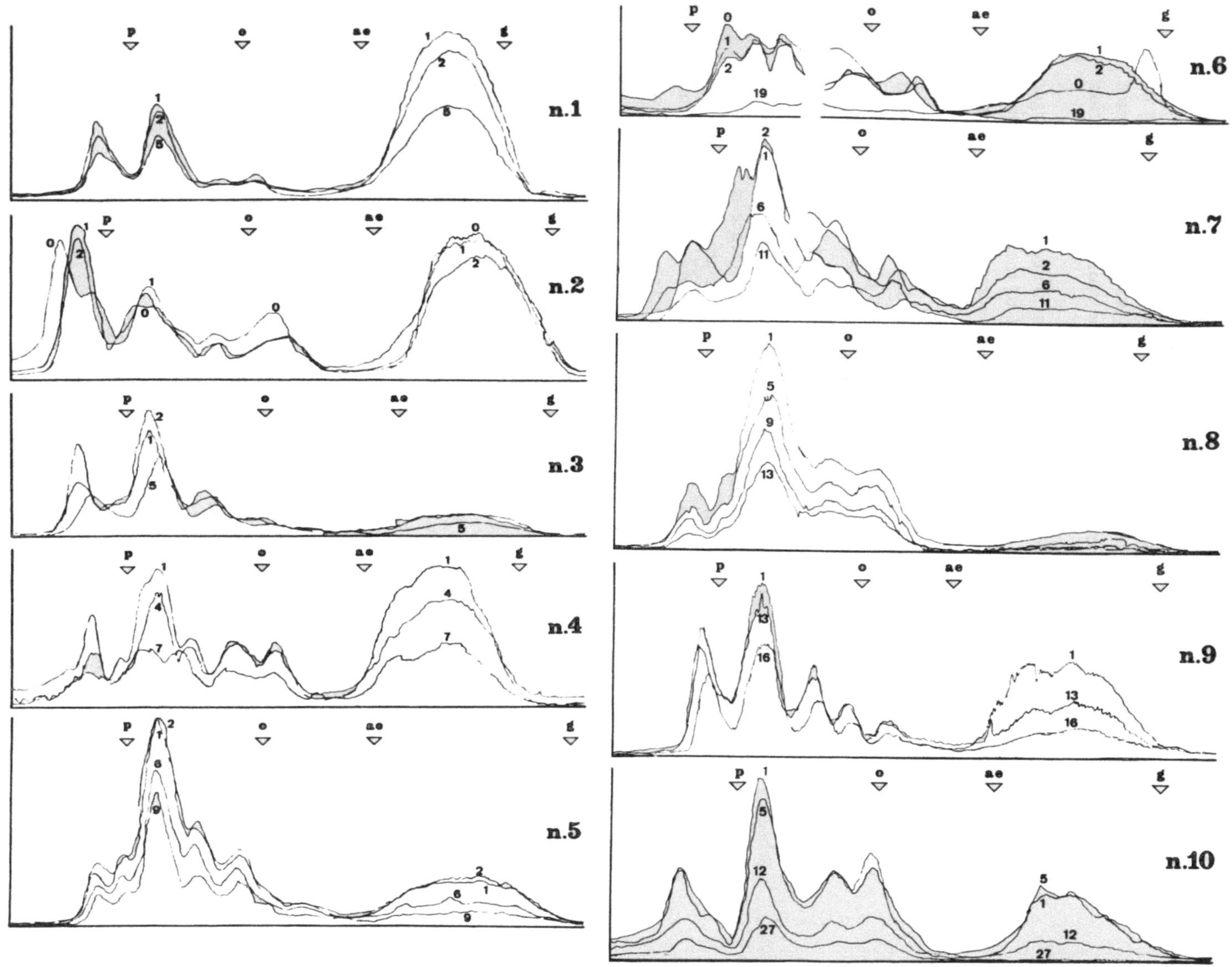

Fig. 4.23. Linear scans (body profiles) for a group of ten patients receiving endolymphatic radiotherapy. The numbers on the curves correspond to the time in days between the injection and the examination. The reference points are indicated by small letters (*p* = pubis; *o* = navel; *ae* = ensiform apophysis; g = neck). As can be seen, in some cases (patients nº 5, 6, 10) there was an increase in radioactivity during the first few days at level of pulmonary area and in other cases (patients nº 2, 3, 5, 7) at the level of the lymph nodes. This difference can probably be attributed to a higher degree of diffusion of the contrast medium from the more distal lymph nodes

each tissue simultaneously exposed to β and γ radiations will receive a dose equal to the sum of the dose due to the β radiation, plus that due to the electromagnetic radiation.

The physical half-life will obviously be the same for both the β and γ radiation, as this is characteristic of the radioisotope.

The distribution of the β and γ rays throughout the human body is conditioned solely by the metabolic processes of absorption and elimination of the ^{131}I.

The distribution of the dose due to the β rays is limited by the finite range of the β rays themselves (a range of the order of a few mm of tissue); hence, the greater part of the dose within and in the immediate vicinity of the radioactive localization will be due mainly to the β particles.

On the contrary the dose due to the γ rays will be distributed through a larger tissue extent, because of the interaction mechanism related to their electromagnetic nature. For this reason, the intensity of the dose due to the γ rays will be influenced considerably less by a non-uniform distribution of the radioactive material than that due to the β rays.

On the other hand, the γ dose absorbed will be strictly dependent, not only on the energy of the electromagnetic radiation in question, but also on the form and dimensions of the tissues that contain the radioisotopes, as well as of the surrounding tissues. Consequently, geometry plays a very important part in the dosimetry.

As mentioned, the β particles bear the greatest responsibility for the dose absorbed by the organ under examination. Usually, when evaluating the dose absorbed by tissues impregnated with β and γ radioactive substances, reference is made only to the β rays. Nevertheless, we will here give the formulas for an exact calculation of the dose taking into account the contribution to the total dose due to both β and γ rays. Then, by means of a scintillation counter connected to a counting system, we can measure the intensity of the flow of γ radiation from the patient treated with labelled lipiodol. In so doing, we can determine how the radioactive substance is distributed throughout the organism, its concentration in the various organs of interest, and the effective half-life of ^{131}I in the different regions (on the basis of the methods described above).

In order to determine the effective half-life (T_e) of the radioisotope in a given organ, one plots on a graph along the ordinate (logarithmic scale) the values of the activities measured at various time intervals, and along the abscissa (natural scale) the time values for the different measurements. Within the limits of the approximations made on the assumption that the concentration (or the activity) has an exponential type behaviour, the result will be a straight line. By extrapolating this line to zero, one can establish the effective regional physical half-life (T_e) as the abscissa of the $\frac{C(o)}{2}$ ordinate point (or $\frac{A(o)}{2}$).

The dose accumulated per gram of tissue, up until the complete elimination of the radioisotope, is calculated (according to data given in the literature) on the basis of the following relations:

$$D_\beta(\infty) = 73.8\, \bar{E}_\beta\, C_0\, T_e \quad \text{rad} \tag{1}$$

$$D_\gamma(\infty) = 0.0346\, \varrho\, \Gamma\, \bar{g}\, C_0\, T_e \quad \text{R} \tag{2}$$

where: $\bar{E}_\beta$ is the average energy of the β rays.

It is defined mathematically as:

$$\bar{E}_\beta = \frac{\int_0^{E_{Max}} E\,N(E)\,dE}{\int_0^{E_{Max}} N(E)\,dE}\ \mathrm{MeV/dis.}_\beta$$

where N (E) is the function that describes, substantially, the trend of the β emission spectrum.

$\bar{E}_\beta$ represents the energy which on the average, for every disintegration can be absorbed by the tissue as a consequence of the radioactive decay that took place within the tissue itself. The $\bar{E}_\beta$ values given in the literature have been obtained experimentally (that is, through graphic integration on the basis of β spectra obtained experimentally), as well as theoretically by using the $N(E)$ expression for permissible spectra deducible from Fermi's theory.

The approximate rule is that $\bar{E}_\beta$ is equal to about one third of the maximum energy (E_{max}) emitted by disintegration.

C_0 is the concentration of radioactive substance at the time expressed as $t=0$.

Assuming for $C(t)$ the expression $C(t)=C_0\,e^{-\frac{0.693}{Te}t}$, one can easily see how, once having determined $C(t)$ according to the previously mentioned methods, it is possible to calculate C_0.

T_e is the effective half-life of the radioisotope in the region under examination and is expressed in days.

ϱ is the density of the radioactively impregnated tissue. (For muscle, ϱ can be assumed to equal 1.)

Γ is the so-called "dose factor", i. e. the intensity of the dose (in R/hr) at a distance of 1 cm from a point source of the radioisotope in question, of an activity equal to 1 mCi: for ^{131}I, $\Gamma = 2.18\ \frac{\mathrm{cm^2 \times R}}{\mathrm{mCi \times hr}}$.

$\bar{g}$ is the "geometric factor".

This latter term takes into consideration the form and dimensions of the organ being considered.

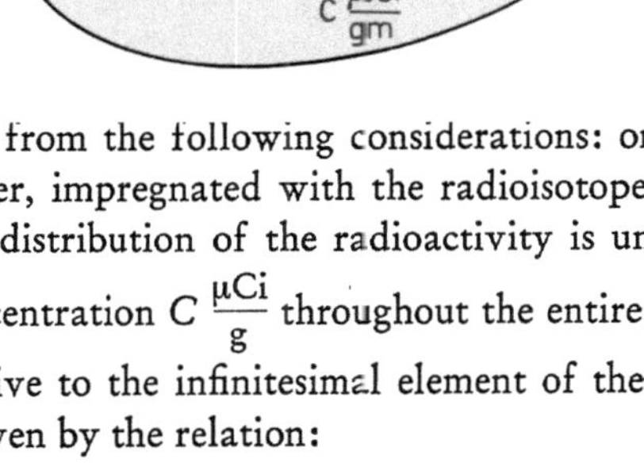

This factor derives from the following considerations: one thinks of a volume V of any form whatsoever, impregnated with the radioisotope in question. One moreover assumes that the distribution of the radioactivity is uniform and constant and characterized by a concentration $C\ \frac{\mu\mathrm{Ci}}{\mathrm{g}}$ throughout the entire volume V. The intensity of the dose at P, relative to the infinitesimal element of the volume, positioned at a distance r from P, is given by the relation:

$$dR_{\gamma,P} = \frac{10^{-3}\,C\,\varrho\,\Gamma\,e^{-\mu_{eff}\,r}}{r^2}\,dV \quad \mathrm{R/hr}$$

where $10^{-3}\, C\, \varrho$ is the concentration of the radioisotope in $\frac{\mu Ci}{g}$; Γ is the previously defined term, and μ_{eff} is the effective absorption coefficient. The total intensity of the dose at P, due to the presence of the radioactivity throughout the volume V, will be obtained by integrating the preceding expression on all of V:

$$R_{\gamma, P} = 10^{-3}\, C\, \varrho\, \Gamma \int_V \frac{e^{-\mu_{eff}\, r}}{r^2}\, dV \qquad R/hr$$

The integral, that appears in this relation is indicated as the "geometric factor", $g_P = \int_V \frac{e^{-\mu_{eff}\, r}}{r^2}\, dV$, for the point P. It is self-evident that this geometric factor has to be defined for every point, in so far as it is a function of the co-ordinates of any point which from time to time may be considered and which varies considerably inside the volume containing the γ emitting substance.

However, in view of the fact that frequently the intensity of the average dose received by the impregnated tissue is more interesting than the intensity of the dose at a single point in a given volume, an average geometric factor can be used:

$$\bar{g} = \frac{1}{V} \int_V g_P\, dV \qquad cm$$

Strictly speaking, this $\bar{g}$ would have different values according to the patient being examined. In practice, we use a value calculated on the basis of the form and dimensions of the same organ in a standard body.

On the basis of what has been stated, equations (1) and (2) can be written in the following way:

$$D_\beta(\infty) = 14\, C_0\, T_e \qquad rad$$

$$D_\gamma(\infty) = 0.075\, \bar{g}\, C_0\, T_e \qquad R$$

Supposing that the dose from the β-particles (in rads) and the dose from the γ-rays (in R) are additive in their biological effect, the total dose will, consequently, be given by the relation:

$$D_{(\beta+\gamma)} = 14\, (1 + 0.052\, \bar{g})\, C_0\, T_e \qquad rad$$

which for specific cases becomes:

lymph nodes $\quad D_{(\beta+\gamma)} = 15\, C_0\, T_e \quad$ rad (*) (1)

thyroid $\quad D_{(\beta+\gamma)} = 16\, C_0\, T_e \quad$ rad (*) (2)

liver $\quad D_{(\beta+\gamma)} = 20\, C_0\, T_e \quad$ rad (*) (3)

spleen $\quad D_{(\beta+\gamma)} = 17\, C_0\, T_e \quad$ rad (*) (4)

entire organism $\quad D_{(\beta+\gamma)} = (25 - 14\, K)\, \frac{A.\,S.}{P}\, T_{1/2} \quad$ rad (5)

where: "A. S." indicates the radioactivity initially injected into the patient; K the fraction retained by the lymph nodes; P the body weight of the patient; and $T_{1/2}$ the decay time deducted from the urinary elimination curve.

In conclusion, the total dose given to the organism, including the lymphatics, is expressed by the formula:

$$D_{tot} = 25\; A.\,S.\; T_{1/2} \qquad grad$$

(*) Besides the various local geometric conditions, the radiations from the source and from the organism in its entirety, have been taken into account.

Acknowledgements

The Author is greatly indebted to Dr. F. di Pietrantoni for his valuable collaboration.

References

Bagliani, G., Buraggi, G. L., de Vecchi, A., Fava, G.: Comportamento della radioattività polmonare in pazienti sottoposti a radioterapia endolinfatica con Lipiodol F ^{131}I. Tumori **53**, 3, 225—236 (1967).

Bertoli, M. A., de Vecchi, A., di Pietrantoni, F., Fava, G., Molese, V.: A contribution to the study of the metabolism of Lipiodol F ^{131}I introduced lymphatically. Medicina Nucleare Radiobiologica Latina **XI**, 2, 167—180 (1968).

Brownell, G. L.: Theory of Radioisotope Scanning. From 'Medical Radioisotope Scanning'. Vol. I. Proceedings of the Symposium on Medical Radioisotope Scanning held by the International Atomic Energy Agency in Athens, 20—24 April 1964. Ed. International Atomic Agency, Vienna, 1964, pag. 3—34.

Buraggi, G., L., d'Amico, P., Fava, G.: La radioterapia endolinfatica. Aspetti tecnici e fisico-biologici. Radiol. med. (Torino) **IL**, 3, 238—273 (1963).

— Fava, G., Roncoroni, L., Agostini, C.: La scansione lineare nello studio delle localizzazioni secondarie dei tumori tiroidei. Medicina Nucleare Radiobiologica Latina. **VIII**, 259—289 (1965).

— d'Amico, P., Fava, G.: La terapia radioisotopica dei linfonodi. Estratto da „Corso superiore di aggiornamento sulla chemioterapia dei tumori“ 7—12 maggio 1962. Ed. Istituto Nazionale Tumori, Milano.

Casiraghi, L.: Tesi di laurea in Fisica „Dosimetria in organi mediante contatori a scintillazione“ 1964—1965.

Cordoni, L.: Tesi di Laurea in Fisica „Dosimetria beta mediante rilevamento dall'esterno dell'intensità di Bremsstrahlung“ 1968—1969.

Craig, C., Bell, P. R., Francis, J. E., Jr., Satterfield, Jordan, J. C., Murray, J. P., Jr.: Collimators for Radioisotope Scanning. From 'Progress in Medical Radioisotope Scanning' Proceedings of a Symposium at the Medical Division of the Oak Ridge Institute of Nuclear Studies, oct. 22—26, 1962. U. S. Department of Commerce, Washington, pag. 25—65.

de Vecchi, A., Bertoli, M. A., Fava, G., Guindani, A., Prada, G., Mazzola, A.: Activity emitted with the expired air by patients subjected to endolymphatic radiotherapy. Medicina Nucleare Radiobiologica Latina **XI**, 4, 329—340 (1968).

— — — Hliniakova: Andamento dell'attività totale e distrettuale nei pazienti sottoposti a radioterapia endolinfatica. Tumori **54**, 2, 221—236 (1968).

Fava, G.: Distribuzione del Lipiodol F ^{131}I nella terapia endolinfatica. Corso superiore sulle malattie mielo-linfoproliferative 129—137, 28. marzo — 2. aprile 1966. Ed. Istituto Nazionale Tumori, Milano.

— Valutazioni dosimetriche nella terapia radioisotopica dei linfonodi con Lipiodol F ^{131}I. Minerva nucl. **7**, 11, 467—472 (1963).

— Il problema della dosimetria nella radio-terapia loco-regionale con isotopi radioattivi. Atti II Simposio Internazionale sul Trattamento regionale dei Tumori, Roma. Minerva med. **58**, 99, 4484—4486 (1967).

— Buraggi, G. L.: A method for the experimental determination of radioisotope concentration in human organs by external counting techniques. Nucl.-Med. (Stuttg.) **III**, 4, 372—381 (1963).

— — Agostini, C., Casiraghi, L.: Scansione lineare: studio analitico e sperimentale dei sistemi di collimazione. Medicina Nucleare Radiobiologica Latina **VIII**, 2, 151—173 (1965).

— Emanuelli, H.: Apparecchiature, tecniche e problemi dosimetrici nella diagnosi e terapia con radioiodio delle metastasi tiroidee. „Corso superiore sulla diagnosi e terapia delle metastasi“. 8—13 maggio 1967. Ed. Istituto Nazionale Tumori, Milano.

FAVA, G., RONCORONI, L.: Body distribution of Lipiodol ^{131}I following Intralymphatic Radiotherapy. Nucl.-Med. (Stuttg.) **V**, 1, 1—11 (1965).

— — Controlli autoptici sulla introduzione nei vari organi del Lipiodol radioattivo, introdotto per via linfatica. Radiol. med. (Torino) **L**, 7, 653—659 (1964).

HEINZEL, F., RÖSLER, H.: Quantitative investigation of the dynamics of intralymphatically applied substances. In: Progress in Lymphology. Ed.: H. RUTTIMAN. Proc. Int. Symp. Lymphology, Zurich 1966. Stuttgart: Thieme 1967.

HERBERT, M., LLOYD, M. D., TIMOTHY STRING, S., ARTHUR, B. A. and B., DU BOIS, M. D.: Radiographic and plethysmographic determination of total lung capacity. Radiology **86**, 7 (1966).

KOEHLER, P. R., WEJERS, W. A., SKELLEY, J. F., SCAGGER, B.: Body distribution of etiodol following lymphangiography. Radiology **82**, 866—871 (1964).

LOEVINGER, R., HOLT, J. G., HINE, G. J.: Internally Administered Radioisoptopes. From 'Radiation Dosimetry'. Edited by G. J. HINE and G. L. BROWNELL. Academic Press Inc., New York, 1956, Chapter 17, pag. 801—908.

PFANNENSTIEL, P., WEISSLEDER, H., HOFFMANN, G.: Problems of radiation dosimetry in endolymphatic therapy with radioactive isotopes. Lymphology **2**, 160 (1969).

— WETZIG, E., KLEINE, N.: Strahlendosimetrie bei der endolymphatischen Therapie mit ^{131}I. In: Radionuklide in Kreislaufforschung und Kreislaufdiagnostik. Hrsg.: G. HOFFMANN, u. R. HOFER. Stuttgart: Schattauer 1968.

— — WEISSLEDER, H., STRICKSTROCK, K. H., KLEINE, N., HOFFMANN, G.: Probleme der Strahlendosimetrie bei endolymphatischer Therapie mit Radionukliden. München: Urban & Schwarzenberg. Sonderband Strahlentherapie **69**, 186—196 (1969).

PICARD, J. D., GONDORA, R., SZIGETI, B., BILSKI-PASQUIER, G., JAMMET, H., ARVAY, N.: Considerations techniques et premiers resultats des injections intra-lymphatiques de Lipiodol radioactif à doses therapeutiques. Ann. Radiol. (Paris) **7**, 543—554 (1964).

POCHIN, E. E.: Profile Counting. From 'Medical Radioisotope Scanning Proceedings of a Seminar jointly organized by The International Atomic Energy Agency and the World Health Organization Vienna, 25—27 February, 1959. I.A.E.A., Vienna, 1959, pag. 143—162.

RATTI, A., CHIAPPA, S., FAVA, G.: I principi e le indicazioni della terapia endolinfatica con Lipiodol F marcato con ^{131}I. Minerva med. **56**, 46, 2013—2015 (1965).

— FAVA, G., RONCORONI, L.: Problemi di diagnosi e terapia radiologica dei tumori della tiroide. Atti della Società Italiana di Cancerologica **5**, 237—310 (1964).

ROSS, D. A.: Linear Scanning. From 'Progress in Medical Radioisotope Scanning'. Proceedings of a Symposium at the Medical Division of the Oak Ridge Institute of Nuclear Studies, oct. 22—26, 1962. U. S. Department of Commerce, Washington, pag. 190—204.

SEITZMAN, D. M., WRIGHT, R., HALABY, F. A., FREEMAN, J.: Radioactive lymphoangiography as a therapeutic adjunt. Amer. J. Roentgenol. **89**, 140—149 (1963).

WEISSLEDER, H., PFANNENSTIEL, P., STRICKSTROCK, K. H., HOFFMANN, G.: Die endolymphatische Therapie mit radioaktiven Substanzen (Technik und Radiometrie). Fortschr. Röntgenstr. **107**, 758—764 (1967).

ZUM WINKEL, K., BECKER, J., JAHNS, E., SCHEURLEN, H., HERZFELD, U.: Indikationsstellung und Dosimetrie bei der endolymphatischen Therapie mit ^{131}J-Lipiodol. Strahlentherapie **133**, 481—498 (1967).

Chapter 5

Clinical Results of Endolymphatic Radiotherapy

S. Chiappa, R. Musumeci, and C. Uslenghi

With 21 Figures

1. Case Material

On the basis of earlier clinical information, from September 1961 to June 1969 we have treated 426 patients by E.R.T. at the National Cancer Institute, Milan. All these patients had biopsy-proven malignant lymphomas in various stages of evolution, as follows: 208 patients with Hodgkin's disease (HD), 95 with lymphosarcoma (LSA) and 123 with reticulum cell sarcoma (RSA).

From September 1961 to April 1964, the majority of patients were treated with E.R.T. but not following strict criteria. E.R.T. was almost always administered to patients in whom the disease no longer seemed to react favourably to the cycles of conventional radiotherapy or to chemotherapy. In the majority of these patients, the disease was therefore at an advanced stage (III and IV). E.R.T. was at first administered to these patients for experimental purposes in small doses (0.2—0.8 mCi/ml) and then in progressively increasing doses up to 2.5 mCi/ml. From May 1964 E.R.T. has been administered in doses of 2.5 mCi/ml in all cases in which the presence of malignant lymphomas has been histologically proved, with the sole exception of cases of LSA and RSA arising from Waldeyer's ring and with adenopathies located in the cervical area (Table 5.1). The total amount of contrast material seldom exceeded a volume of 10 cc for each foot.

The injection of Lipiodol ^{131}I, that is a radio-opaque contrast material, is used both for diagnostic examination and as a therapeutic or prophylactic tool when the lymph nodes are well opacified.

Every case was evaluated 24 hours after the injection of contrast medium through antero-posterior lateral and oblique films. Follow-up films were taken every 2 to 6 weeks, according to the various clinical situations, as long as the contrast material was visible on the radiograph (average 5—8 months, occasionally even one or two years). A second injection of Lipiodol ^{131}I was carried out in 30 patients (20 with HD and with LSA or RSA), either because a retroperitoneal node recurrence was suspected or evident on the follow-up films, or when systemic signs and symptoms occurred without clinical and/or radiological evidence of lymphomatous lesions.

Our abundant case material has enabled us to make several clinical considerations.

Table 5.1. *Number of patients treated per year with minimal and maximal doses of Lipiodol* ^{131}I

Year	Hodgkin's disease		Lymphosarcoma Reticulum cell sarcoma	
	No. cases	Dose mCi/ml	No. cases	Dose mCi/ml
1961	4	0.4—1.7	2	0.2—0.8
1962	25	0.5—2.0	24	0.6—1.8
1963	15	1.7—2.8	10	1.4—2.5
1964	20	2.0—2.5	27	1.9—2.5
1965/69	144	2.5	155	2.5
Total	208		218	

2. Value of Lymphography in the Staging of Patients

Of 426 lymphographies with Lipiodol ^{131}I, 410 were performed in patients with primary lymph-node involvement and 16 in patients in whom the lymphoma had arisen in other primary sites, outside the lymph nodes.

Table 5.2 gives the incidence of lymph node abnormality for every stage of various histological types of malignant lymphoma, expressed in percentages. The clinical staging was determined after completion of recommended studies, with the exception of lymphography. It is apparent from this table that, in patients staged

Table 5.2. *Abnormal lymphograms in 410 malignant lymphomas with primary lymph node involvement*

Clinical staging	Hodgkin's disease		Lymphosarcoma		Reticulum cell sarcoma	
	No. cases	Abnormal lympho-grams %	No. cases	Abnormal lympho-grams %	No. cases	Abnormal lympho-grams %
I_1	42(3) [a]	36	20(2) [a]	55	19	45
I_2	32(1) [a]	68	8(1) [a]	38	13	50
II	81(2) [a]	65	11(1) [a]	60	14	65
III	21	84	33	98	31	80
IV	31	90	18	100	36	70
Total	207		90		113	

[a] In brackets the number of patients with primary onset below the diaphragm.

Table 5.3. *Abnormal initial lymphograms in 16 untreated malignant lymphomas with primary extranodal involvement*

Primary site	Hodgkin's disease		Lymphosarcoma		Reticulum cell sarcoma	
	No. cases	Abnormal lymphograms	No. cases	Abnormal lymphograms	No. cases	Abnormal lymphograms
Stomach			2	0	4	3
Small intestine					1	0
Skin			2	2	1	0
Bone	1	0			3	0
Parotid			1	1		
Maxillary antrum					1	0
Total	1	0	5	3	10	3

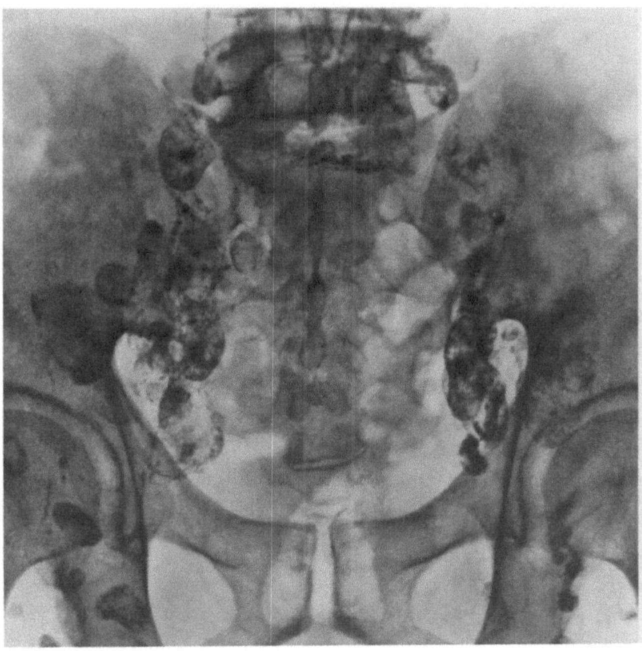

Fig. 5.1. Male, 49 years old. For 3 months fever, night sweats and abdominal pain. All clinical and X-ray investigations were negative. Follow-up film 24 hours after E.R.T. — The retroperitoneal lymph nodes appear typically pathologic. Retroperitoneal biopsy = Hodgkin's disease

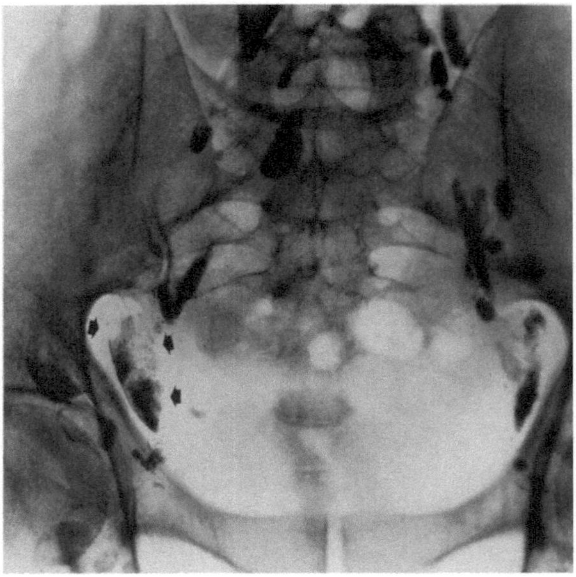

Fig. 5.2. Male, 53 years old. Hodgkin's disease, clinically stage I_1 (left cervical area). Follow-up film 24 hours after E.R.T. = A lymph node in the right iliac chain (arrows) shows typical lacunar filling defects. A biopsy confirmed the lymphographic diagnosis. This patient was classified after E.R.T. as stage III

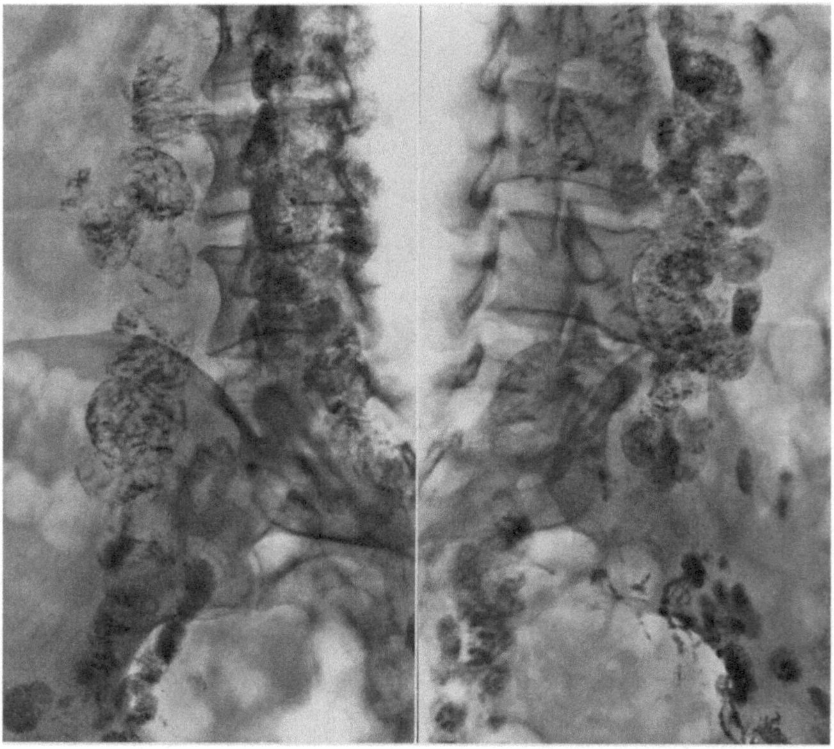

Fig. 5.3. Female, 68 years old. Reticulum cell sarcoma arising from Waldeyer's ring, clinically stage I_2. Follow-up film 24 hours after E.R.T. Lymphographic polymorphism of pathological retroperitoneal lymph nodes. This patient was classified after E.R.T. as stage III

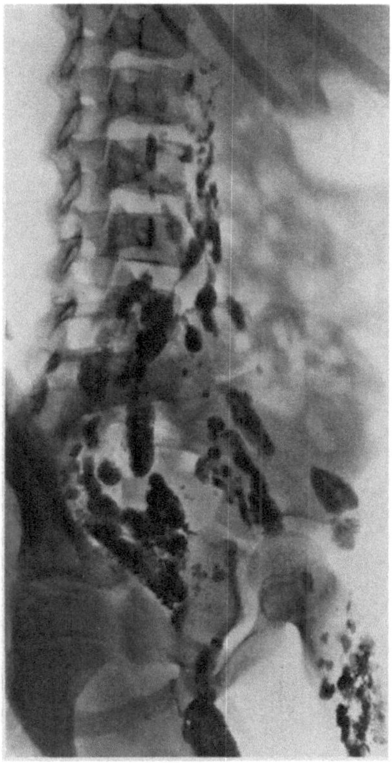

Fig. 5.4. Girl, 4 years old. Histologically proven lymphosarcoma of the small bowel and spleen. Follow-up film 24 hours after E.R.T. Pathologic lymph nodes in the right iliac area

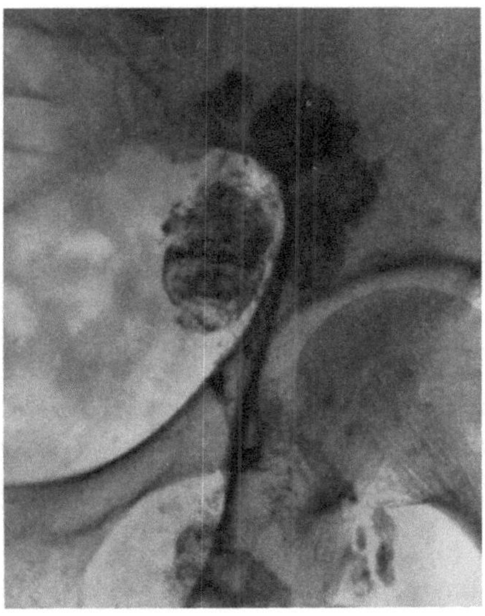

Fig. 5.5. Female, 49 years old. Lymphosarcoma of the right parotid gland. Follow-up film 24 hours after E.R.T. Pathologic lymph nodes in the left iliac chain. Iliac biopsy = LSA

as I_1, the lymph nodes of the retroperitoneal chains were involved in 36% of the cases with HD, in 55% of the cases with LSA and in 45% of the cases with RSA. In the patients staged as I_2, the data are 68%, 38%, 50% respectively; in the patients staged as II, the involvement was greater (65%, 60%, 65%), and still

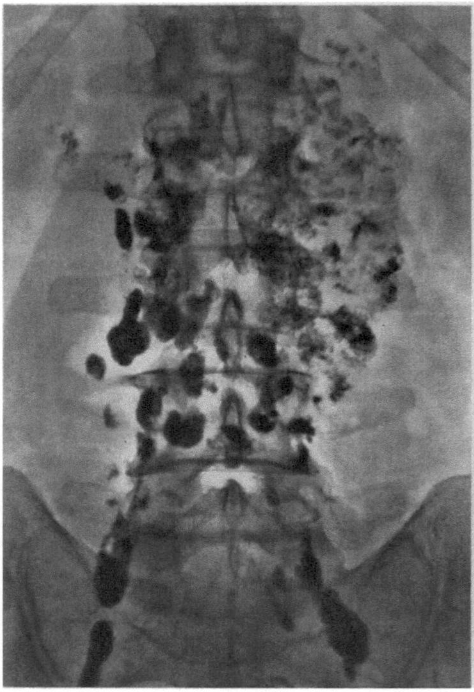

Fig. 5.6

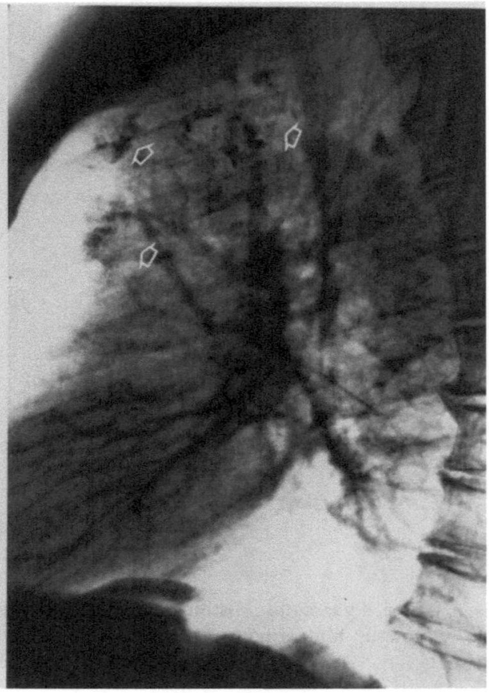

Fig. 5.7

Fig. 5.6. Male, 40 years old. Reticulum cell sarcoma clinically only above the diaphragm (Stage II). Follow-up film after E.R.T. Pathologic lymph nodes in the para-aortic area, especially on the left side. The patient was classified after E.R.T. as stage III

Fig. 5.7. Same case. Lateral chest film. Several mediastinal lymph nodes are opacified with ^{131}I Lipiodol and appear invaded by the disease (arrows)

greater in cases staged as III (84%, 98%, 80%) or IV (90%, 100%, 70%). In some cases staged as III, lymphography was negative and there was only involvement of the spleen.

Table 5.3 shows the results of radioactive lymphograms in 16 malignant lymphomas with primary extranodal involvement: pathological nodes were detected in the retroperitoneal area in 3/6 cases with gastric LSA or RSA, in 2/2 cases of LSA of the buttock and in one case of primary LSA of the parotid gland.

The results of this study, in a large number of cases, confirm that there is a high incidence of silent retroperitoneal adenopathies in cases of malignant lymphoma clinically classified as in the initial stages of the disease, and that there is a progressive increase in the number of cases with retroperitoneal involvement in HD going from stage I_1 to stage II, whereas in LSA and in RSA the involvement is more irregular. (Figs. 5.1, 5.2, 5.3, 5.4, 5.5).

In a small number of cases, lymphography was able to opacify pathologic mediastinal lymph nodes. (Figs. 5.6, 5.7, 5.8).

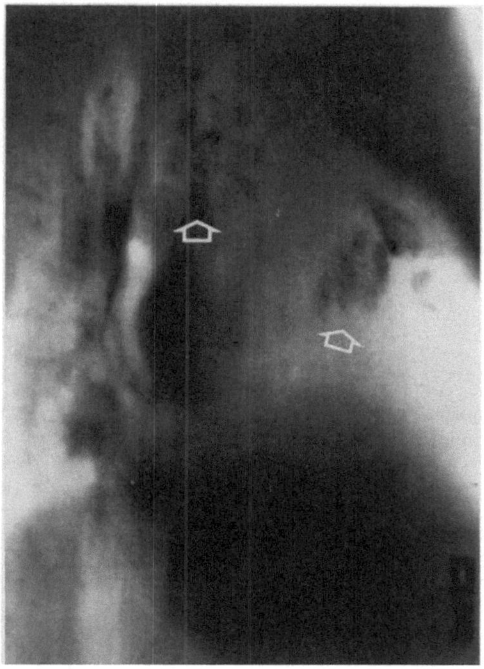

Fig. 5.8. Same case. Lateral tomogram of the chest. Clearer evidence of the involved mediastinal lymph nodes (arrows)

3. Factors Preventing a Complete and Homogeneous Distribution of Radioactive Contrast Material

We should like to point out at once that the use of this technique is subject to limiting factors that can considerably impair its effectiveness, whilst it is essential that certain fundamental conditions should be present to obtain useful therapeutic action. This fact is universally recognized and is one of the limitations of lymphography, and, therefore, also of E.R.T. These factors are easily appreciated and can be summarized as follows: first of all, it is indispensable that the lymphatic vessels afferent to the lymph centres have a clear lumen; secondly, there should be a good distribution of the radiating agent within the lymphatic tissue involved.

As Lipiodol is also a contrast medium for lymphography, the X-ray films obtained, both during the vascular phase and the subsequent adenographic phase, enable us to judge how the distribution of the lipiodol, and of the ^{131}I with it, proceeds in the lymph nodes that are to undergo irradiation. It should be borne in mind that the radiation deriving from the disintegration of the ^{131}I which is useful for therapeutic purposes is the beta radiation, having an average energy of 0.5 MeV and a range of 3 mm. This confirms the necessity for uniform impregnation of the lymph nodes.

Table 5.4. *Factors making for uneven distribution of radioactive contrast medium and numbers of patients affected*

Factor	Lymphatic chains	No. Patients
Lymphography not feasible in one foot		27
Extravasation in soft tissues		5
Lymphatic block	Iliac	2
	Para-aortic	4
Bypass	Iliac	4
Abnormal	Inguinal	3
Lipiodol/lymphnode ratio	Iliac	8
	Para-aortic	64
	All chains	18
Total		135 (32.4%)

Table 5.4 shows the patients in whom filling of the lymph nodes with radioactive contrast medium has not given the best results and the reasons for this. In 27 cases, it was not possible to perform lymphography from one foot owing to difficulty in finding a lymphatic vessel with a suitable lumen for cannulation. This has usually occurred in children, in young adults and in patients with conspicuous edema due to varicosities. In 5 patients, an extravasation of the contrast medium into the soft parts surrounding the injection site was observed; this seems to be due to excessive pressure when injecting and to unexpected movements made by the patient causing breakage of the lymphatic vessel. As will be explained in more detail further on, spillage of ^{131}I into the soft tissues generally does not have side effects worthy of note. In 6 cases, a blockage of the lymphatic way was reported, namely, in one case of HD and in 5 cases of LSA or RSA (Fig. 5.9). In 4 patients with HD a by-pass of the iliac nodes took place.

All the side effects described above occurred in 42 patients. In a much larger number of cases [93], an uneven distribution of the contrast material in the lymph nodes was observed with poor impregnation in some cases. This phenomenon has been observed especially in the region of the para-aortic chains (64 cases), whilst the inguinal and iliac nodes usually became opacified in a satisfactory manner.

It is, therefore, evident that the distribution of the radioactive contrast material has not taken place evenly in 135/426 patients, or 32.4%. This is due, as we have already mentioned, to various causes, both technical and of an other nature. The

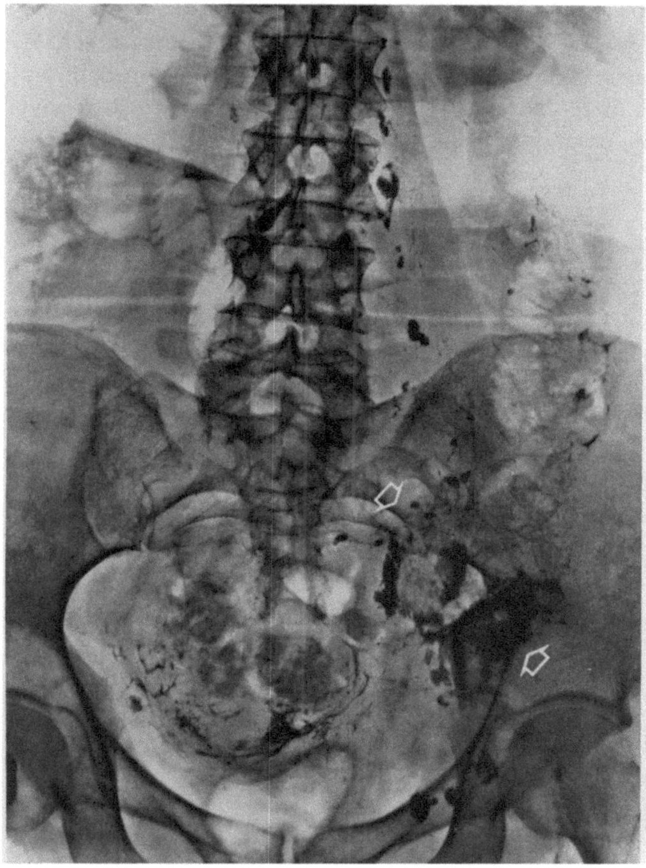

Fig. 5.9. Female, 79 years old. Lymph node swellings in the left iliac area and systemic symptoms for 8 months. Follow-up film 24 hours after E.R.T. from the left foot. Spillage of the ^{131}I Lipiodol in a large necrotic cavity (arrows). Blockage of the lymphatic way in the common iliac chain. Collateral lymph circulation (perivesical plexus, mesocolon lymphatic plexus). Inguinal biopsy = LRSA

fact that the lymph node chains (especially those of the para-aortic area) do not become homogeneously and completely opacified is, in our opinion, the most consistent obstacle to radiotherapy administered correctly and with uniform dosage. This happens most often in HD which, as we have already mentioned, involves mostly the para-aortic chains. For this reason, when the retroperitoneal lymph nodes have not been adequately opacified, we completed treatment with cobalt teletherapy (T.C.T.) (Fig. 5.10).

4. Contraindications

The experience we have acquired with E.R.T. in a large number of patients has enabled us to establish the contraindications to the use of this method of treatment. As a preliminary concept, we feel justified in stating that there are no contraindications of a general nature, as ^{131}I has been administered to patients in whom the disease was widespread without appreciable consequences. The only caution that should be exercised in the administration of ^{131}I is in respect of patients with a systemic disease in the advanced stages with considerable hepatic involvement, as we have in a few cases observed a further deterioration in the liver function tests.

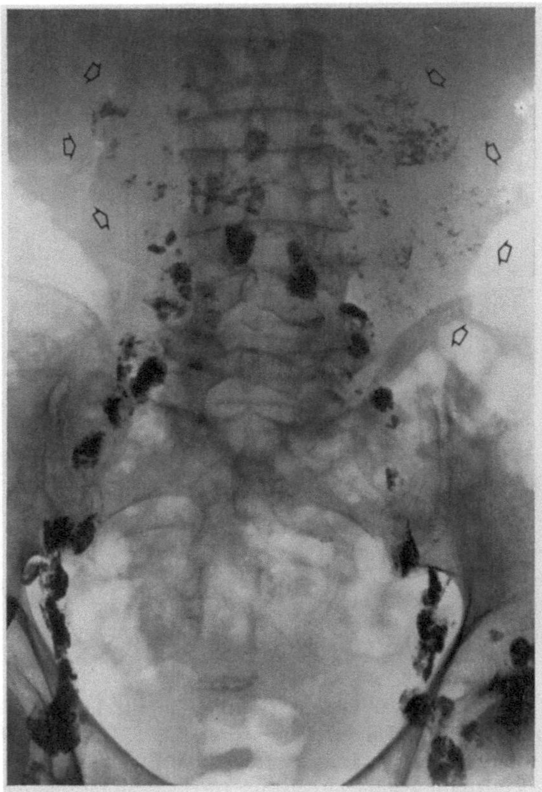

Fig. 5.10. Male, 57 years old. Biopsy-proven LRSA, clinically stage II. Follow-up film 24 hours after E.R.T. Large adenopathies in para-aortic area, very poorly opacified with ^{131}I Lipiodol (arrows). The patient, classified after E.R.T. as stage III, received a course of external T.C.T. (inverted Y field) below the diaphragm

The most important contraindications are certainly the local ones and, of these, the most relevant is lymphatic edema of the limbs. This condition is rarely found in patients with lymphomas, but is relatively frequent in patients with epithelial neoplasia in the pelvis, with involvement of the retroperitoneal lymph nodes by metastases. In the few cases of patients presenting with lymphatic edema, an injection of ^{131}I was in fact given in an attempt to reduce the edema by unblocking the lymphatic collectors and by reducing the dimensions of the adenopathies through the action of the radioactive Lipiodol. In a certain number of cases, the size of the edema decreased considerably within a short period of time, whilst in others no results were obtained and the contrast liquid overflowed into the soft parts.

A second local contraindication is evident in cases treated by external radiotherapy, especially in the inguinal region. In these patients, sclerosis of the lymph-node tissue had set in and the contrast material could not penetrate into the parenchyma of the lymph nodes. Sometimes a similar alteration was observed in the lymphatic collectors too. In view of these considerations, we think it advisable to administer E.R.T. prior to transcutaneous radiotherapy. When this is not possible, we prefer to abstain from treatment with ^{131}I and carry out a diagnostic lymphography.

5. Immediate Clinical Results

We have gathered under this heading all clinical observations on the effects of E.R.T. with regard to the symptoms and signs manifested by our patients.

In some cases it has been observed that the patient's painful abdominal symptoms subsided, these symptoms being obviously due to pressure in the nerve roots or on the various viscera caused by the lymph-nodes swelling. This action is clearly correlated with the local effect of E.R.T. on the lymph-nodes. When the pain ceases, usually the patient's fever drops and the itching also subsides from the first few days after treatment. Therefore, we feel justified in stating that this method of treatment also acts upon the so-called systemic signs when the most conspicuous involvement is in the retroperitoneal space.

The most obvious effect—and hence easier to ascertain—is, however, the striking reduction in the volume of the nodal masses. In some patients, this reduction is clearly manifest from the first few days after the endolymphatic injection of Lipiodol ^{131}I. It is obvious that the reduction in volume takes place more rapidly when the lymph nodes are well opacified by the contrast material. It should, however, be noted that this reduction in volume has been found in all patients who have undergone this type of treatment, even in cases in which the impregnation did not prove to be very good.

6. Radiographic Results

The simplest criterion, and at the same time the most effective in establishing the effect of E.R.T. on systemic adenopathies, is that based on radiographic follow-up at intervals over a period of time. We have already mentioned the follow-up scheme we usually adopt (see chapter A), which must obviously be adjusted in each case according to the clinical evaluation of the disease. The effect of E.R.T. on the lymph nodes, which is clinically appreciable in some cases, as we have already seen, is naturally easier to detect in the X-ray follow-ups (which are, of course, all carried out under the same technical conditions). In fact, when a reduction in the volume of the pathological lymph nodes is found on palpation at the time of the check-up, the lymph nodes opacified by the radioactive contrast material appear even more clearly reduced in size on the X-ray.

The radiographic finding constantly evidenced is thus clearly outlined: the lymph nodes grow progressively smaller in size, with variations that can already be detected a few days after the E.R.T., and this reduction in size continues over a period of 2—3 months, until the lymph nodes practically return to their original size. As time goes by, the lymph nodes lose their opaqueness increasingly owing to spontaneous reabsorption of the contrast material. However, they can still be studied more than 6 months after the introduction of Lipiodol ^{131}I into the lymphatic

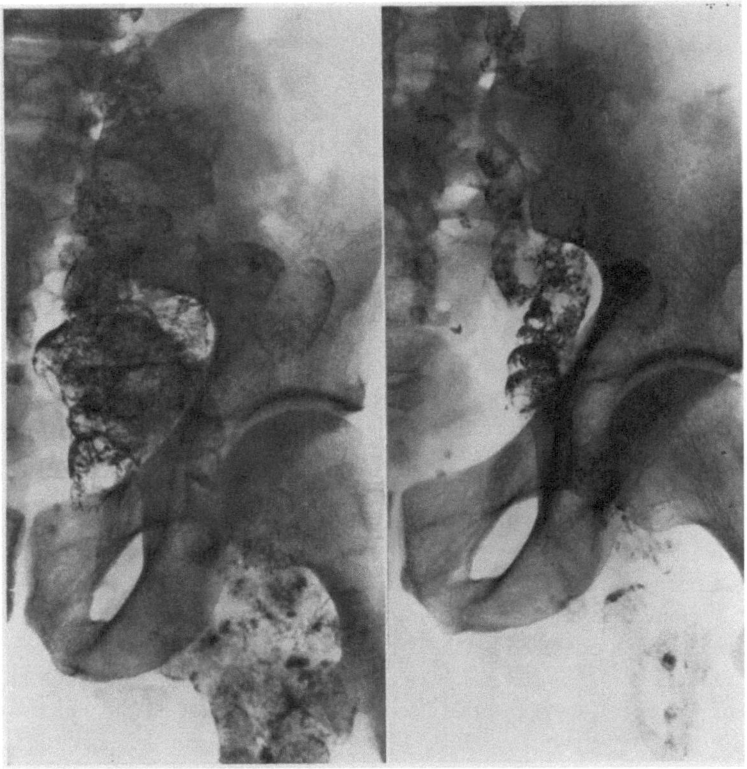

Fig. 5.11 a Fig. 5.11 b

Fig. 5.11 a. Male, 23 years old. Hodgkin's disease with primary onset below the diaphragm. Enormous lymph node swellings in the inguinal and iliac chains

Fig. 5.11 b. Same case. Follow-up film 50 days after E.R.T. Good shrinkage of all opacified lymph nodes

system. Ascertaining the variations in size of the nodes is made easier by the fact that, in some of the cases we handle, the outline of the individual lymph nodes, even where these are affected by the pathological condition, is generally recognizable for a longer period of time, since the contrast material collects mostly in the marginal cavities of the lymph nodes. In cases where the Lipiodol ^{131}I causes a conspicuous and rapid reduction in the dimensions of the lymph nodes, these become even more opaque through the concentration of the contrast material in a smaller volume, thus facilitating check-ups by enabling one to make them over a longer period of time (Figs. 5.11 a—b, 5.12 a—b, 5.13 a—b, 5.14 a—b).

Fig. 5.12 a

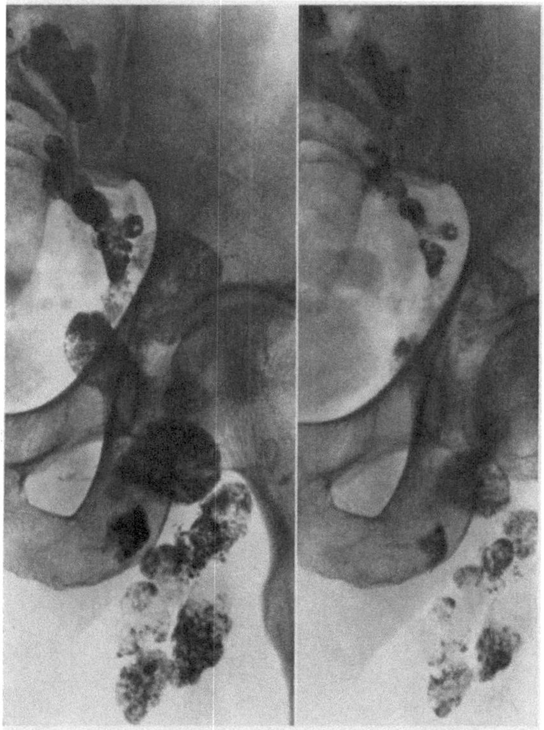

Fig. 5.12 b

Fig. 5.12 a. Female, 27 years old. Lymphosarcoma, clinically stage III. Well opacified lymph nodes, involved by the disease, in the inguinal and iliac chains

Fig. 5.12 b. Same case. Follow-up film 35 days after E.R.T. Good shrinkage of the pathologic nodes

Fig. 5.13 a

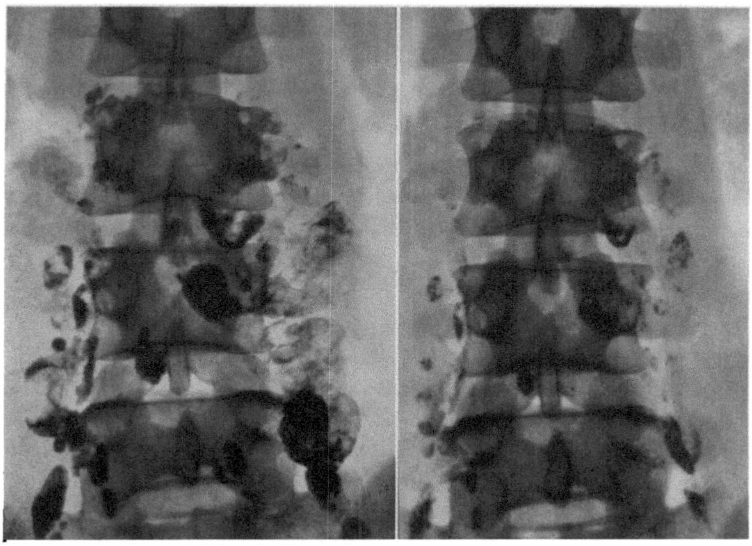

Fig. 5.13 b

Fig. 5.13 a. Female, 18 years old. Hodgkin's disease, stage II (before E.R.T.). Bilateral involvement of the para-aortic node chains

Fig. 5.13 b. Same case. Follow-up film 60 days after E.R.T. Good shrinkage is evident

Follow-up films become particularly important in patients who show clinical signs of a recurrence in the evolution of the disease and in whom a relapse or a new localization in the retroperitoneal chains is suspected. The radiographic signs on which the diagnosis is based consist essentially in an increase in the dimensions of the lymph nodes that should still be partially under the influence of the radioactive Lipiodol, in their shifting further away from the spine (in both a lateral and posterior-anterior direction), in a dislocation of the kidney towards the exterior, in

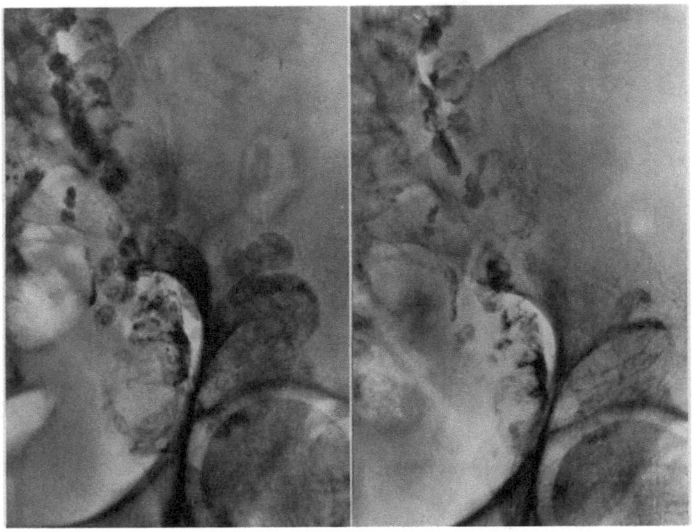

Fig. 5.14 a Fig. 5.14 b

Fig. 5.14 a. Male, 20 years old. Hodgkin's disease, stage III. All the opacified lymph nodes are involved by the disease. Iliac nodes are poorly opacified

Fig. 5.14 b. Same case. Follow-up film 28 days after E.R.T. Though poorly opacified, the iliac lymph nodes appear to have shrunk

an enlargement of the area where the residual traces of Lipiodol that initially appeared closer together owing to the reduction in volume of the lymph nodes have become scattered. It is obvious that signs of relapse or of new localizations of the disease are difficult to diagnose in many cases and only the experience acquired by observing a large number of radiographs can enable one to work along the lines that will lead to the correct diagnosis. In controversial cases which have, however, sufficient grounds to be clinically suspect, a second lymphographic examination may be carried out either with Lipiodol F or with Lipiodol ^{131}I (Figs. 5.15 a—b, 5.16 a—b, 5.17 a—b, 5.18 a—b).

In some cases treated with E.R.T. and having clinical signs of progression of the disease in other body regions, a second injection was performed. In such cases we can see the action of E.R.T. on the opacified lymph nodes. In the films taken during the lymphographic phase, the lymphatic channels are normal in calibre. In the adenographic phase no residual lymph nodes are seen (Fig. 5.19 a—d).

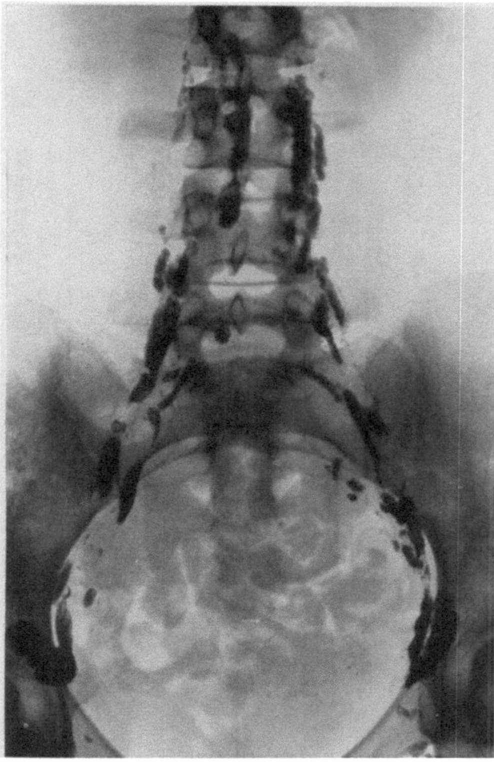

Fig. 5.15 a

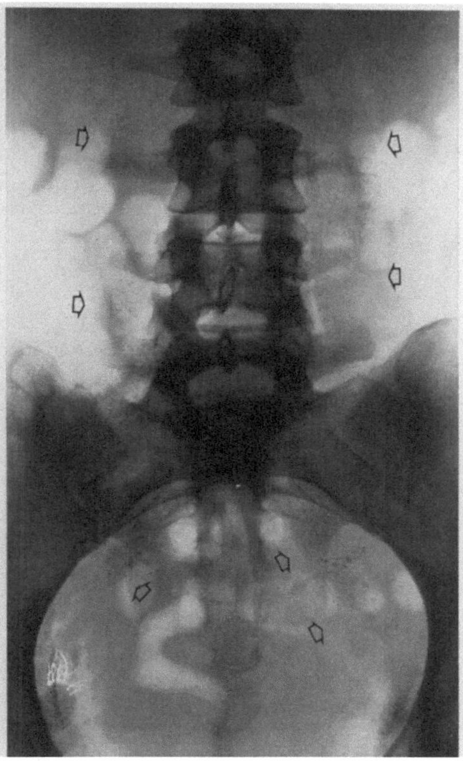

Fig. 5.15 b

;. 5.15 a. Female, 24 years old. Biopsy proven LS A, stage I_2. Follow-up film 24 hours after E.R.T. Retroperitoneal lymph nodes are adequately filled do not appear involved by the disease

g. 5.15 b. Same case. Follow-up film 22 months after E.R.T. New localizations of the disease in all the retroperitoneal chains (arrows)

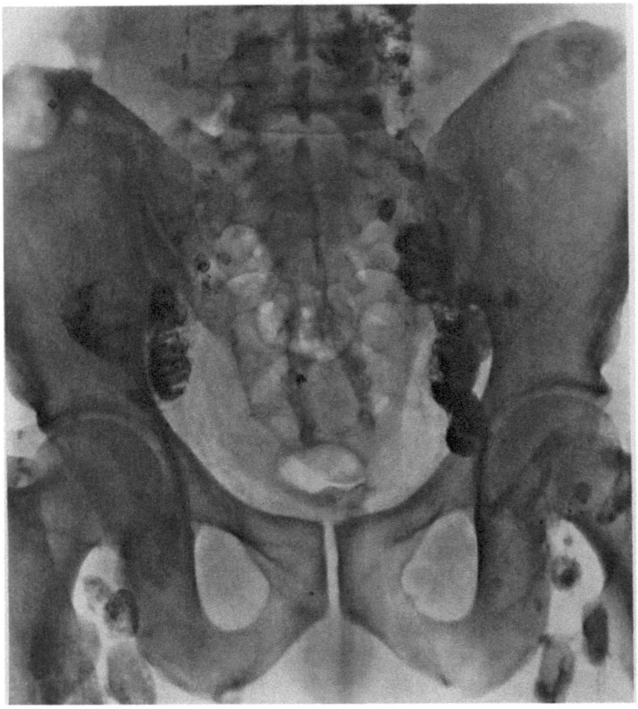

Fig. 5.16 a. Male, 45 years old. Biopsy-proven LRSA, stage III. Follow-up film 24 hours after E.R.T. All the opacified lymph nodes appear involved by the disease

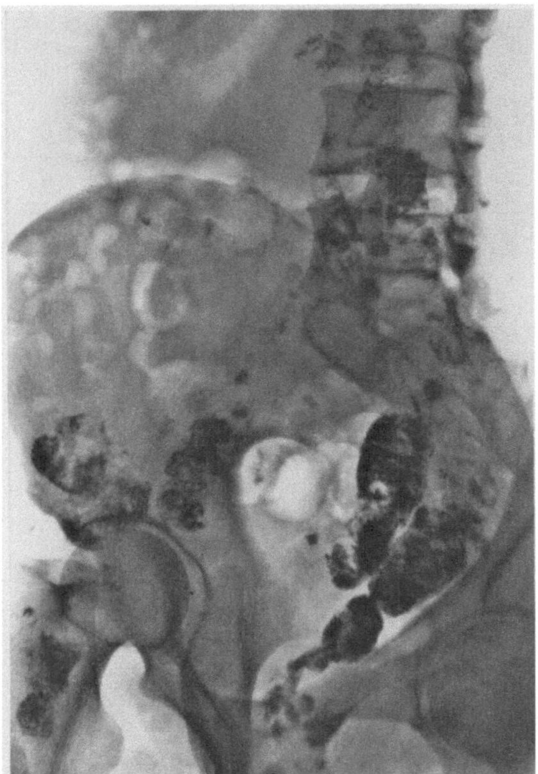

Fig. 5.16 b. Same case: oblique view. Poor filling of the para-aortic node chains is evident

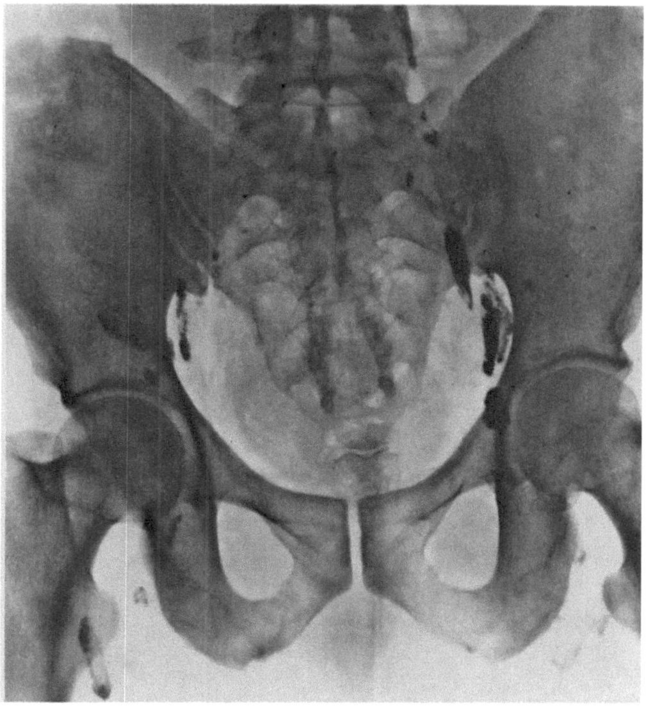

Fig. 5.17 a. Same case as in Figure 5.16 a—b. Follow-up film less than 5 months after E.R.T. Good shrinkage of the opacified lymph nodes of the inguinal and iliac chains

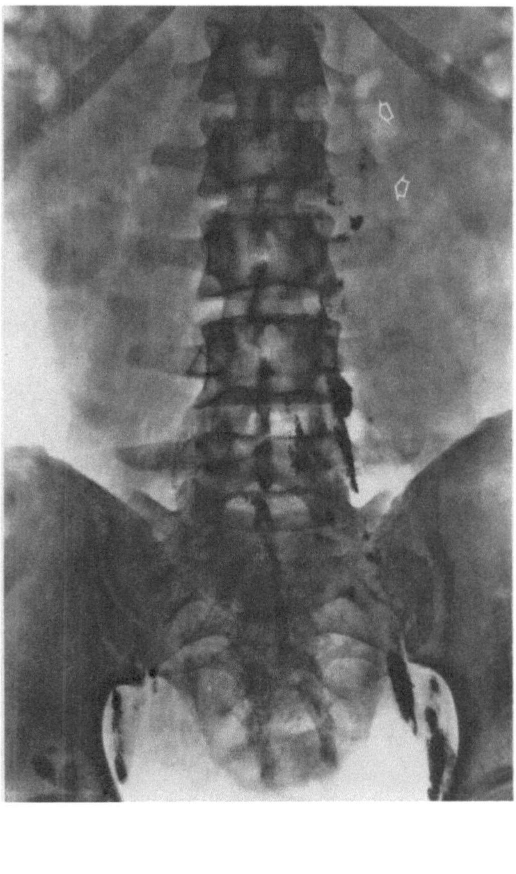

Fig. 5.17 b. Follow-up film of the para-aortic chains in the same patient. Good shrinkage of the lymph nodes though opacified. Pathologic nodes in the left upper side (arrows). A course of external T.C.T. in the para-aortic region was administered

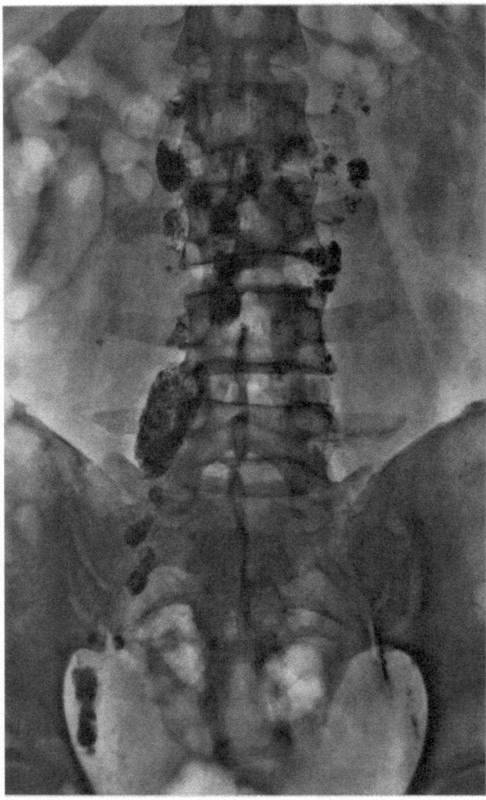

Fig. 5.18 a

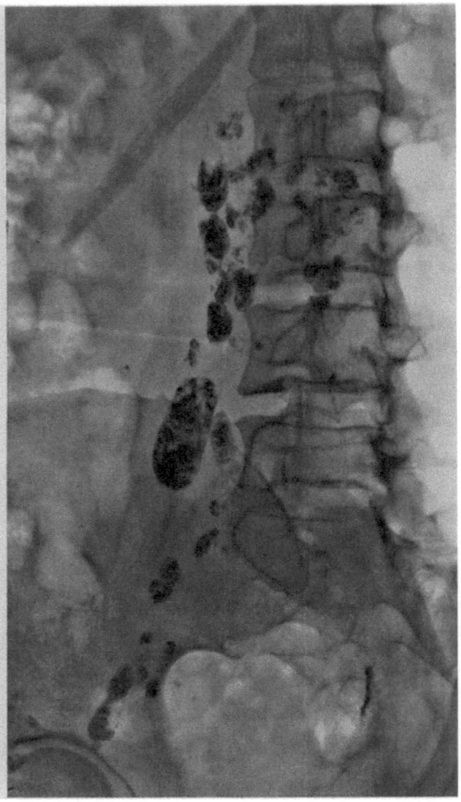

Fig. 5.18 b

Fig. 5.18 a. Same patient as in figures 5.16 a—b and 5.17 a—b. New injection of ^{131}I Lipiodol about 5 years later for systemic symptoms. Recurrence of lymphoma in both sides of the para-aortic area. The iliac chains are not involved. (12. 5. 1969)

Fig. 5.18 b. Same patient; oblique view

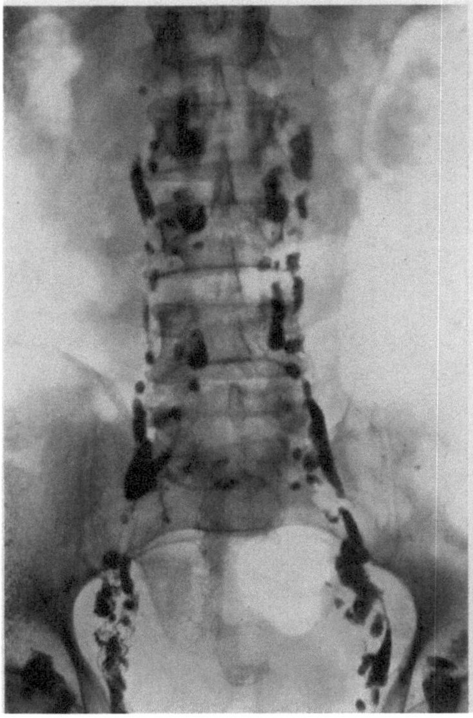

Fig. 5.19 a

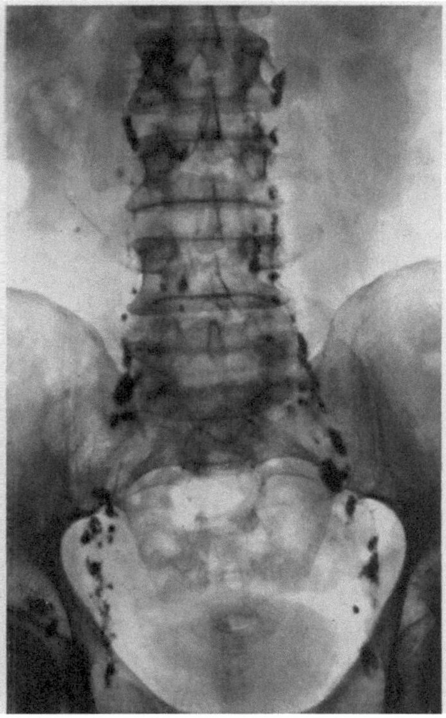

Fig. 5.19 b

Fig. 5.19 a. Male, 48 years old. Biopsy proven LSA, stage I_2. Follow-up film 24 hours after E.R.T. The retroperitoneal lymph nodes are adequately opacified and not involved by the disease

Fig. 5.19 b. Same patient. Follow-up film 46 days after E.R.T. Good shrinkage of all the opacified lymph nodes

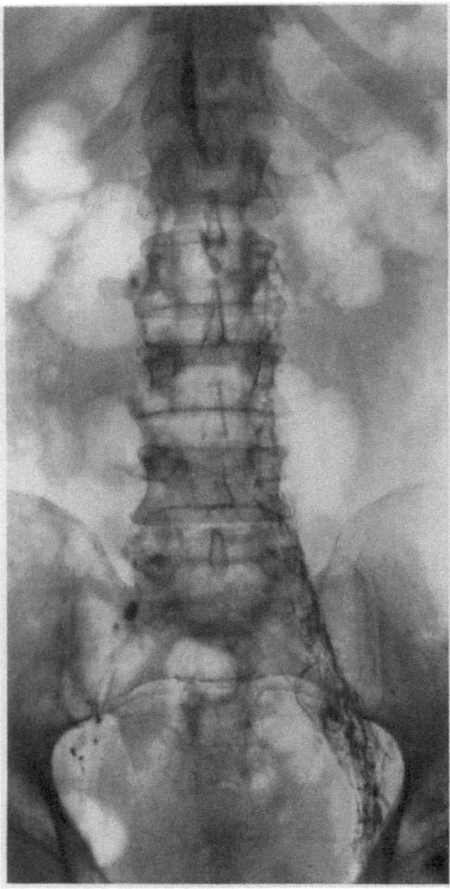

Fig. 5.19 c

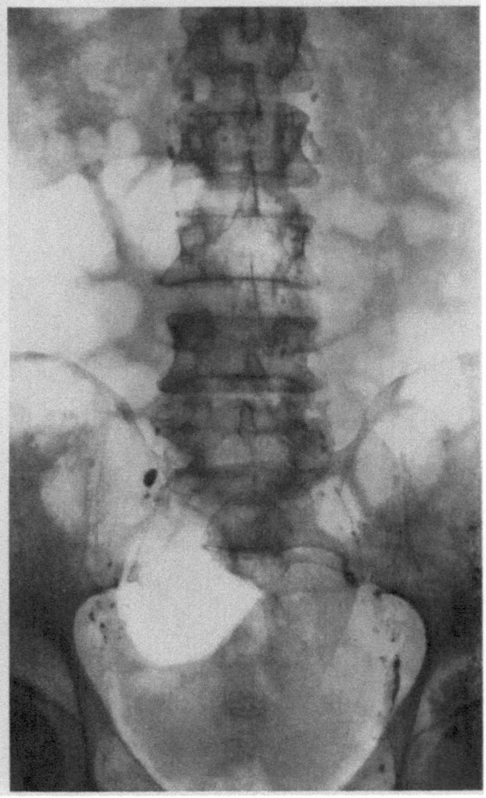

Fig. 5.19 d

Fig. 5.19—c. Same patient. New injection of ^{131}I Lipiodol 3 years later for systemic symptoms. The injection was performed only in the left side. Film taken at the end of the injection. The lymphatic channels appear normally canalized

Fig. 5.19 d. Same patient. Follow-up film 24 hours after the second injection of ^{131}I Lipiodol. No residual lymph nodes are seen in the retroperitoneal area: lymphatic tissue was destroyed by the first injection of ^{131}I Lipiodol

7. Long-term Results. Recurrences and New Localizations of Lymphomas in the Retroperitoneal Chains

The group of patients with various types of malignant lymphomas that have undergone E.R.T., as already mentioned, comprises 426 cases: 36 of these underwent treatment less than 6 months before this review and have not therefore been taken into consideration in drawing up the results. The remaining 390 cases are patients who received E.R.T. during the period from 1st September 1961 to 31st December 1968 and whose follow-up is up-to-date to July 1969 (thus, the observation period ranges from a minimum of 6 months to approximately 8 years).

With regard to the long-term results of this radiotherapeutic treatment, we deem it advisable, when analysing results to consider separately, on the one hand, patients classified in the first stages of the disease (I_1, I_2, II) after lymphography and therefore having a negative lymphogram, and, on the other hand, patients classified in the more advanced stages and therefore having involvement of the retroperitoneal node chains to a greater or lesser extent. As a parameter of the efficacy of this treatment, we have considered a recurrence of the disease in the region of the opacified lymph nodes.

In Table 5.5 these occurrences are analysed separately according to the type of disease and the clinical stage in relation to the time of outbreak. This analysis has been made in patients treated exclusively by E.R.T. (335 patients) in the region of the lymph node chains below the diaphragm; therefore, we have ruled out 55 cases who received external T.C.T.

Table 5.5. *Numbers of patients with recurrence or new localization of the lymphoma in retroperitoneal chains treated with Lipiodol* ^{131}I

		Months after Lipiodol ^{131}I						
Type of lymphoma	Stage	0—6	7—13	14—20	21—27	28—34	35—41	60
Hodgkin's disease	I_1				1	1		
	I_2							
	II							
	III [b]	2	3	3	3	4		
	IV [b]	1			1			
Lymphosarcoma and reticulum cell sarcoma	I_1						1	
	I_2	1 [a]			1			
	II			1 [a]				
	III [b]	2	6	3		1	1	2
	IV [b]					1		
	Other Primary		1				1	
Total (41 patients)		6	10	7	6	7	3	2

[a] Primary onset of disease below the diaphragm.

[b] Patients in these stages had one more courses of chemotherapy and of external radiation therapy above the diaphragm.

Table 5.6. *Number of recurrences or new localizations found in 41 patients and reported in relation to the different lymph node chains, the initial lymphographic findings and the dose of Lipiodol ^{131}I administered*

Type of lymphoma	Lymph node chains	No. recurrences	Lymph nodes at first lymphogram: Normal		Abnormal		Dose of Lipiodol ^{131}I (mCi/ml)		
			AF [a]	IF [b]	AF [a]	IF [b]	0.4—0.9	1.0—1.9	2.0—2.5
Hodgkin's disease	Inguinal	1			1				1
	Iliac	3	1		2			2	1
	Para-aortic	13	3		9	1	1	2	10
	All chains	2			2		1		1
		19	4		14	1	2	4	13
Lympho-sarcoma	Inguinal	10	1		8	1		2	8
	Iliac	8			6	2	2	1	5
	Para-aortic	2	1			1			2
	All chains	3	1		2		2	1	
		23	3		16	4	4	4	15
Total		42	7		30	5	6	8	28

[a] AF = adequately filled with Lipiodol ^{131}I.
[b] IF = inadequately filled with Lipiodol ^{131}I.

Out of 335 patients treated solely by E.R.T., sometimes (stages III and IV) in addition to cycles of chemotherapy, we were able to find 41 patients with a recurrence of the disease or with a new outbreak of the disease in the region of the lymph nodes below the diaphragm (12.2%). In the group of patients in the first two stages, in whom E.R.T. could be considered a "precautionary irradiation", this occurred in only 6 cases. In the more numerous group of patients with a positive lymphography, a relapse occurred at varying intervals of time in 35 cases. Forty-two cases of relapse or of new localization were later confirmed in 41 patients (in one patient the disease broke out again in non-contiguous sites) through X-rays (follow-up films, new injection of Lipiodol, urography, pneumoretroperitoneum, study of the gastro-intestinal tract) and physical examination.

These 42 cases are shown in Table 5.6 in relation to the various lymph node chains, at the first lymphographic examination and at the doses of Lipiodol ^{131}I administered. As can be easily seen from the table, the relapses or new localizations of the disease in the retroperitoneal chains occurred, especially in HD, in the para-aortic chains (13/19 cases, i.e. 69%) and, in LSA or RSA, in the inguino-iliac regions (18/23 cases, i.e. 78%). This bears out our knowledge of "the natural history" of these diseases and of their preferential sites of localization (see chapter 1). Recurrences and progressions were found usually in adequately opacified lymph nodes (37/42 cases) and after high doses of Lipiodol ^{131}I.

On the basis of our experience, the finding of 6 patients with a new retroperitoneal localization is very significant, inasmuch as this figure is low. This could, in fact, indicate that E.R.T. has definite prophylactic value, although it will not be possible to attribute a definite statistical value to it for a long time to come.

A fairly logical explanation of the mechanism by means of which relapses or new localizations occur in the lymph node chains treated by E.R.T. is that some lymph nodes affected by the systemic disease are by-passed by the contrast material

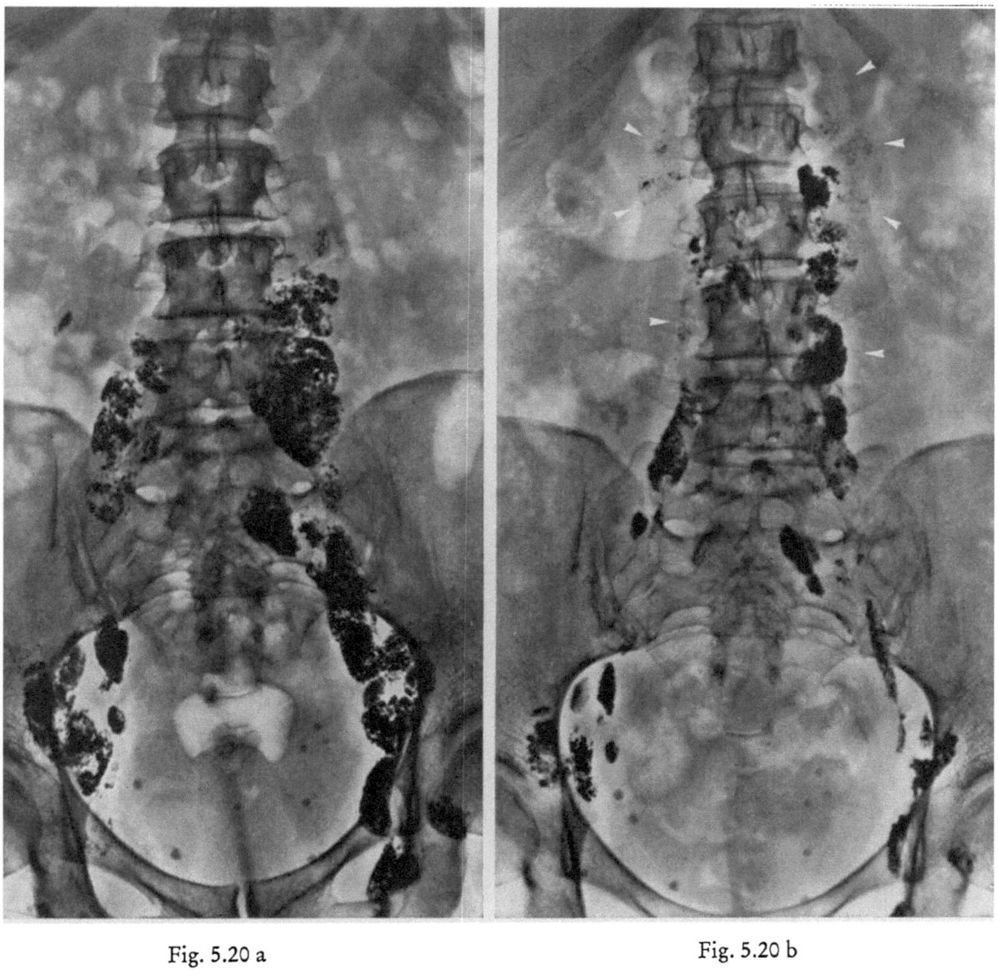

Fig. 5.20 a Fig. 5.20 b

Fig. 5.20 a. Female, 41 years old. Biopsy-proven LRSA, stage III. Follow-up film 24 hours after E.R.T. All the opacified lymph nodes appear involved by the disease. Poor filling of the para-aortic chains. A course of external T.C.T. was administered in this area

Fig. 5.20 b. Same patient: new injection 2 years later for retroperitoneal recurrence (diagnosis after excretory urogram). Follow-up film 24 hours after E.R.T. Recurrence in the para-aortic area (arrows), treated with external T.C.T. The iliac chains treated only with E.R.T. appear not to be involved and therefore escape irradiation. Another interpretation is based on the uneven distribution of the Lipiodol ^{131}I within the lymph nodes affected by the lymphomatous process, causing incomplete destruction of the neoplastic tissue and having a residue of lymphoma cells that are free to proliferate and cause a new outbreak of the disease.

Purely by way of an example, we would like to report the restricted group of 55 patients in whom E.R.T. treatment was completed by means of a course of transcutaneous T.C.T. In Table 5.7 we show cases of relapse or failure to recover

Table 5.7. *Number of patients showing recurrence or progression after treatment with external radiation therapy to lymph node chains inadequately filled with Lipiodol* ^{131}I

Type of lymphoma	Stage	No. cases	Recurrences (months)				
			0—6	7—13	14—20	21—27	28—34
Hodgkin's	III [b]	25		2	1		
disease	IV [b]	9	1				
Lymphosarcoma	I_2	1 [a]			1		
retaculum cell	III [b]	13		1			
sarcoma	IV [b]	7		1			
		55	1	4	2		0

[a] Primary onset of disease below the diaphragm.
[b] Patients in these stages had one or more courses of chemotherapy and of external radiotherapy above the diaphragm.

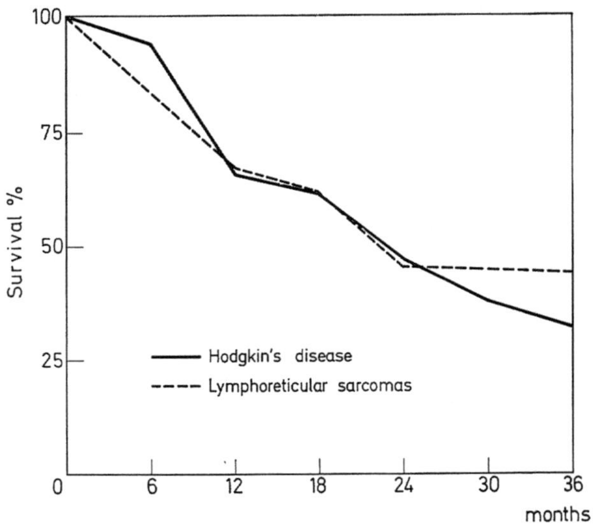

Fig. 5.21. Three-year survival rate in malignant lymphomas classified after E.R.T. as stage III. These patients received external T.C.T. above the diaphragm and courses of chemotherapy. The retroperitoneal chains were treated only by E.R.T.

after treatment by T.C.T. of the retroperitoneal lymph node chains not adequately opacified after E.R.T. and involved in the lymphomatous process (stages III and IV). In this limited group of patients the number of relapses was 7 (12.7%) (Fig. 5.20 a—b).

The task of ascertaining data from our case material proved arduous as, it turned out that note of the patients were treated exclusively with E.R.T. during the whole course of the disease. Many patients, in fact, received courses of chemotherapy and radical or palliative treatment with T.C.T. above the diaphragm. Research in this connection has revealed results that perhaps cannot be estimated clinically, but that we have thought advisable to consider for guidance purposes. It has been possible to establish the survival rate (within the limitations mentioned above) in patients classified as stage III after lymphography, as they represent the largest group. In this group we have found a survival rate of 48% at 3 years, in cases of LSA and RSA, and of 37% in HD. On the basis of our experience, these results are remarkably good, in spite of the influence that other types of therapy undoubtedly have on the progress of the disease.

References

For references on this chapter, see Chapter 2.

Chapter 6

Side Effects and Complications

S. Chiappa, R. Musumeci, and C. Uslenghi

With 11 Figures

A variety of complications and side effects have been reported by all investigators working on diagnostic lymphography and E.R.T. It is, however, evident that those caused specifically by E.R.T. should be considered separately from the others as regards their causes and importance [1—2, 6, 8—9, 13—14, 20—23, 25—26].

Table 6.1. *Side effects and complications of endolymphatic radiotherapy with Lipiodol* ^{131}I

Side effect or complication	Hodgkin's disease	Lymphoreticular sarcomas
Extravasation necrosis	2	1
Lymphangitis	1	2
Hyperthyroidism	1	
Hepatic insufficiency	2	
Pulmonary insufficiency	2	1
Hemolytic anemia	1	
Amenorrhea	12/75 [a]	2/35 [a]

[a] Menstruating females.

Table 6.1 shows the complications and side effects that have arisen following the systematic use of E.R.T. in 426 patients. As can be seen, complications and side effects have been found in 27 out of 426 patients, or about 6.3%. Local complications, such as necrosis caused by spillage of the radioactive contrast material into the soft tissues or ascending lymphangitis, have been observed in only 6 patients (Figs. 6.1, 6.2, 6.3). These complications, although not very important from a clinical point of view, should always receive attention because they can cause considerable discomfort to the patient. However, in all our cases, they have been controlled by appropriate therapy. In some cases edema of one or both legs follows lymphography or E.R.T. (Fig. 6.4) [29]. In order to avoid such side effects, we usually monitor on a television screen the rise of the radioactive contrast material in patients who have previously undergone inguinal biopsy or have had courses of external radiotherapy to the inguinal regions, so as to stop the flow of the Lipiodol ^{131}I at the first signs of spillage. It is in patients in this group that surgical intervention or sclerosis of

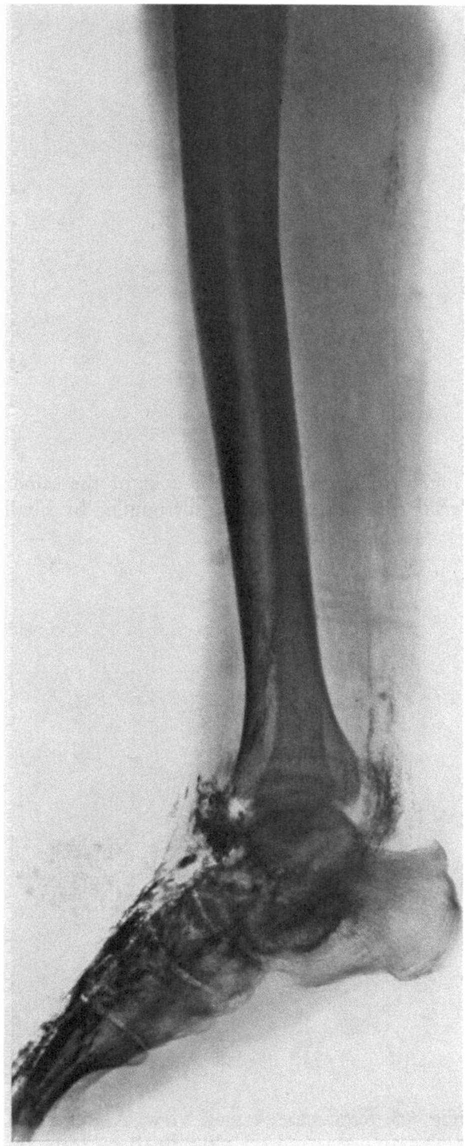

Fig. 6.1. Follow-up film 24 hours after lymphography. The film shows abundant spillage of the radioactive contrast medium (Lipiodol ^{131}I) in the soft tissues of the dorsum of the foot, of the ankle and of the calf

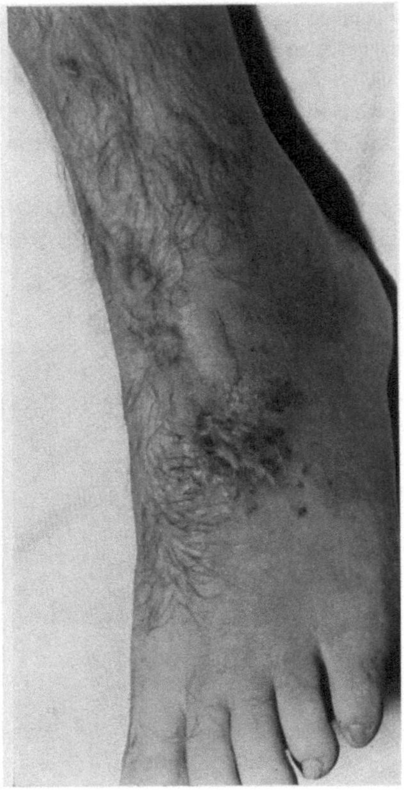

Fig. 6.2. Photograph of the foot of the same patient 120 days after E.R.T. The surgical incision did not heal and is surrounded by small necrotic areas. The soft tissues are oedematous

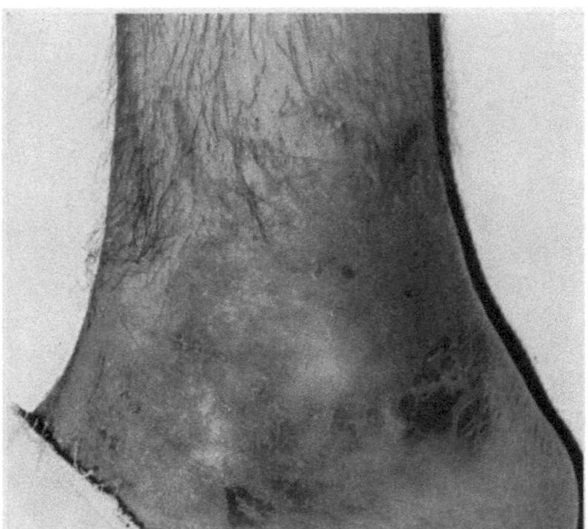

Fig. 6.3. Same case: lateral view. Are clearly seen the oedema of the soft tissues of the ankle, the small necrotic areas and the loss of hairs

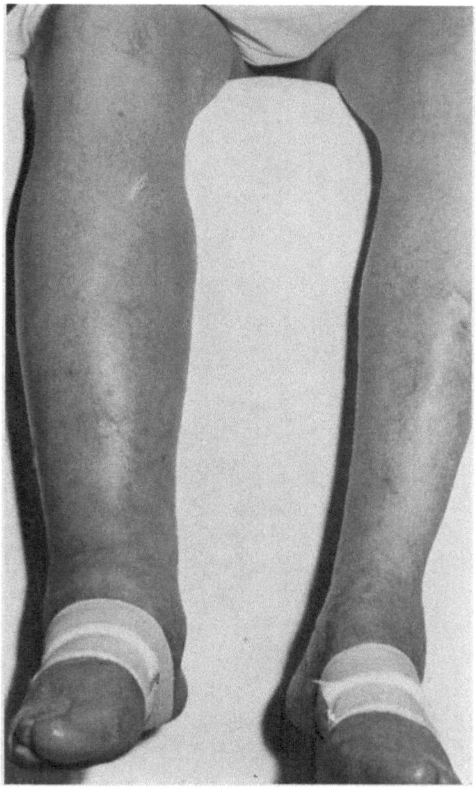

Fig. 6.4. Photograph of the legs of a patient 60 days after E.R.T. Conspicuous oedema of the right leg, ankle and foot. The left foot is oedematous while the left leg appears to be normal. The surgical incisions did not heal

the lymphatic collectors caused by radiotherapy tend to produce stasis at the root of the limb with formation of a collateral circulation, lymphatic ectasia and increase of parietal fragility. In some patients in whom partial lymphadenectomy of the inguinal lymph nodes was carried out for biopsy purposes, we were able to observe and document radiologically the formation of lymphatic pseudocysts of varying dimensions in which the contrast material collects (Fig. 6.5). In such cases, when the contrast material is radioactive and a relatively large quantity is present, a high degree of irradiation in neighbouring territories ensues and radionecrosis may set in (Figs. 6.6 and 6.7).

Scintiscan studies have proved that radioactive Lipiodol accumulates in the thyroid in doses that vary between 1500—2000 rad. These doses are undoubtedly very high and, therefore, a potential source of disorders of a hypothyroid nature. Although no patients with hypothyroidism were seen in our case material, as can be seen from the table, but only one isolated and unaccountable case of hyperthyroidism, we would recall that the administration of Lugol drops in the days preceding the radioactive lymphography can "block" the thyroid, preventing the accumulation of ^{131}I and the subsequent unwanted irradiation [30].

In our experience, which includes autopsy, no cases of cerebral embolism from Lipiodol ^{131}I have been observed: two such cases are reported by other investigators [7, 28].

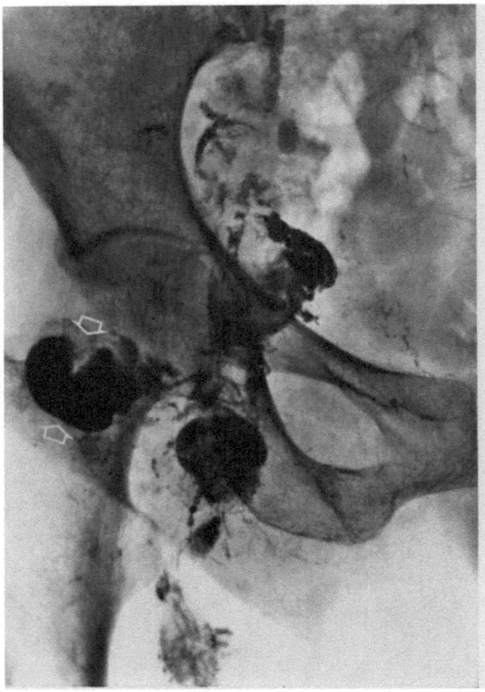

Fig. 6.5. Follow-up film 24 hours after lymphography in a patient with Hodgkin's disease. The patient has previously undergone inguinal biopsy. At the site of the biopsy incision the formation of a lymphatic pseudocyst is clearly seen (arrows)

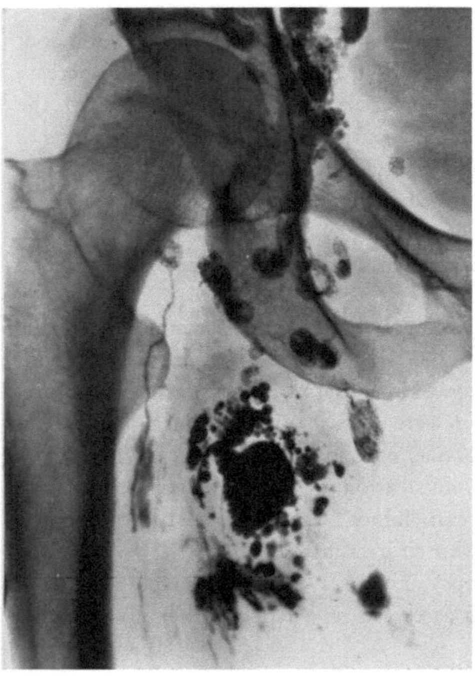

Fig. 6.6. Follow-up film 24 hours after lymphography in a patient with reticulum cell sarcoma. The patient had previously undergone inguinal biopsy. At the site of incision one can observe the formation of a lymphatic pseudocyst and the diffusion of droplets of Lipiodol ^{131}I in the surrounding soft tissues

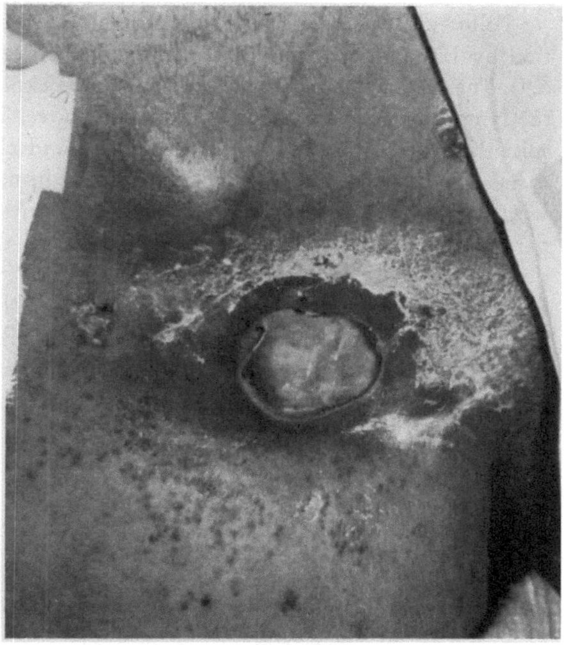

Fig. 6.7. Photograph of the same patient 50 days after E.R.T. At the site of the lymphatic pseudocyst is a large (2×3 cm) ulcer with an indurated and elevated edge. All around the central ulcer there are many small necrotic areas and oedema of the soft tissues. This ulcer is certainly due to radionecrosis

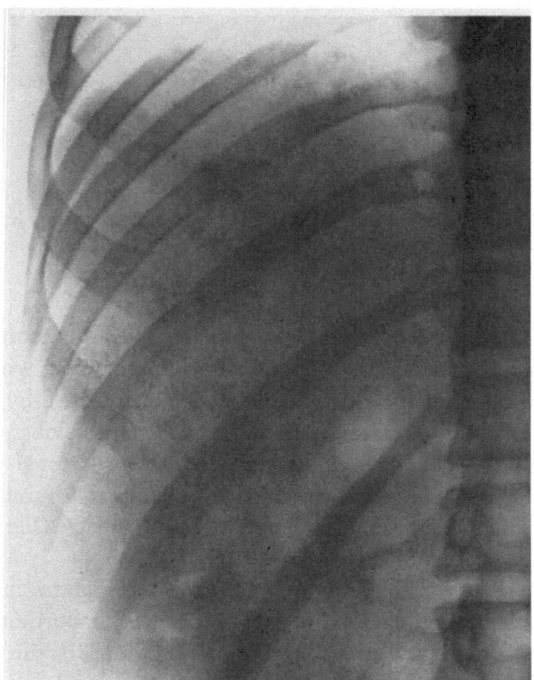

Fig. 6.8. Film of the right upper abdomen 24 hours after lymphography in a patient with Hodgkin's disease. Hepatic impregnation of Lipiodol ^{131}I is clearly seen with the typical pattern of thin arborized stripes

Following E.R.T., it has been possible to recognize on X-rays hepatic impregnation by Lipiodol in two cases and splenic impregnation in one case (Figs. 6.8 and 6.9). The mechanism leading up to this can be explained by taking into consideration the lympho-venous anastomoses described above. The case with impregnation of the spleen has been followed up radiologically and clinically for about two years, but it has not been possible to find any clinical, hematologic or biochemical alterations worthy of note or, at all events, connected with the impregnation of the splenic parenchyma and its irradiation at high doses. In the two cases of hepatic impregnation, the patients concerned had Hd at stage IV with conspicuous hepatic involvement. The impregnation was followed by signs of hepatic insufficiency with jaundice, markedly elevated direct and indirect serum bilirubin, and high serum levels of SGOT and SGPT. These patients died within a few days with signs of massive hepatic necrosis [31].

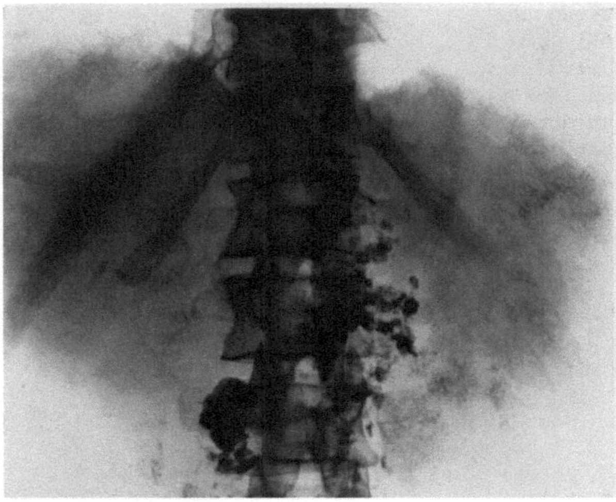

Fig. 6.9. Follow-up film 24 hours after lymphography in a patient with lymphosarcoma. Splenic, hepatic and probably kidney impregnation by Lipiodol ^{131}I. Dissemination of small radiopaque spots

All investigators who have studied diagnostic and radioactive lymphography have reported that pulmonary impregnation with Lipiodol is frequently observed radiologically. This phenomenon is manifested by well-known findings, namely, very thick dissemination, especially in the lower lobes, of slightly radiopaque spots which give the lung an appearance defined as "frosted glass". All authors, however, agree that the radiologic findings of pulmonary infarction are very rarely associated with clinical findings of pulmonary insufficiency (Fig. 6.10) [1—4, 6, 8—9, 11—23, 25 to 26, 32—34].

The quantity of Lipiodol that accumulates in the lungs is variable and depends on different factors, of which the most important have proved to be excessive pressure when injecting, the use of Lipiodol UF, the presence of lympho-venous anastomoses and the disproportion between the volume of the retroperitoneal lymphonodal tissues and the quantity of contrast material injected. In cases in which the embolism can be documented, a re-absorption of the iodized oil within a maximum of 4—7 days has been observed radiographically. In cases in which ^{131}I has been used, scintiscan studies have shown an accumulation of radioactive material in the lungs in quantities that vary in individual cases but are constant, also in patients with a completely negative chest film. This radioactivity decreases rapidly in about two weeks and is practically not measurable after about one month.

Signs of pulmonary insufficiency have been found in three of our patients: in all three cases a conspicuous mediastinal and pulmonary parenchymal involvement was present (two cases of HD and one case of RSA). In these cases, immediately after the injection, the patients complained of severe dyspnea with cyanosis and of dry cough. The radiographic and scintigraphic studies showed that a conspicuous

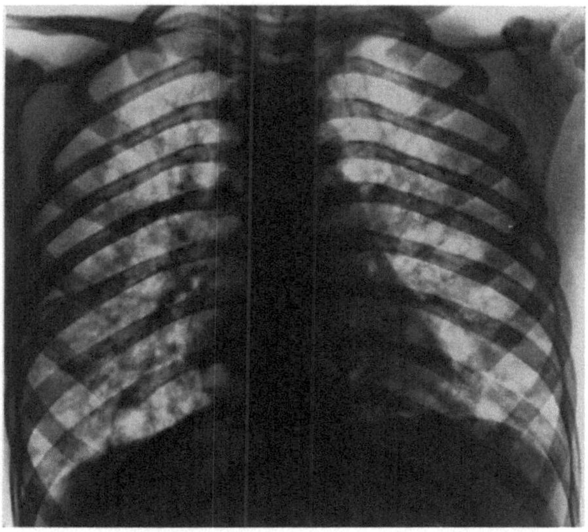

Fig. 6.10. Chest film 24 hours after lymphography in a 10-year-old patient with Hodgkin's paragranuloma. Thick dissemination of slightly radiopaque shadows, especially in the lower lobes, partially confluent. The "frosted glass", appearance is evident

accumulation of Lipiodol ^{131}I was present in both lungs. One of the two patients with HD died about one week later owing to bronchial and pulmonary infections, whilst in the other two cases the patient's condition gradually returned to normal within a few days. Sometimes, even in the absence of pulmonary infarction, low-grade fever is reported the day after the lymphography. This fever, on which antibiotic treatment has little effect, is of unknown genesis (pyrogens in the dye, in the anaesthetic, or in the contrast material?) and generally disappears very rapidly.

At this point, we think it useful to emphasize that, in cases in which a post-mortem examination of the patient was made at varying periods of time after E.R.T., very careful histological examinations of the liver and the lungs at periodic intervals showed no parenchymal injuries attributable in any way to E.R.T. (see Chapter 7).

In one patient with HD, 24 hours after E.R.T., jaundice with high indirect bilirubin, anaemia and reticulocytosis was found; direct Coomb's test proved to be negative. In this case, hemolytic anaemia was diagnosed and a high blood level of ^{131}I was found which persisted for about one week. In this patient, a standard total dose of 20 ml of Lipiodol F ^{131}I was administered, and a very sparse filling of the retroperitoneal lymph nodes involved by the disease was found, as well as a modest pulmonary impregnation evaluated only by scintiscan. In this case it is very likely that some lympho-venous anastomoses were open. It is our opinion, according to the postulate of Lewis et al., that in this case ^{131}I probably acted as a "trigger mechanism" [27].

Another side effect found in our case material is amenorrhea, observed in 14 patients out of 110 at a fertile age (12.7%). The E.R.T. acts through direct irradiation of the ovary which in some cases may result from, large iliac lymph node masses that collect a large quantity of radioactive material. In the majority of cases,

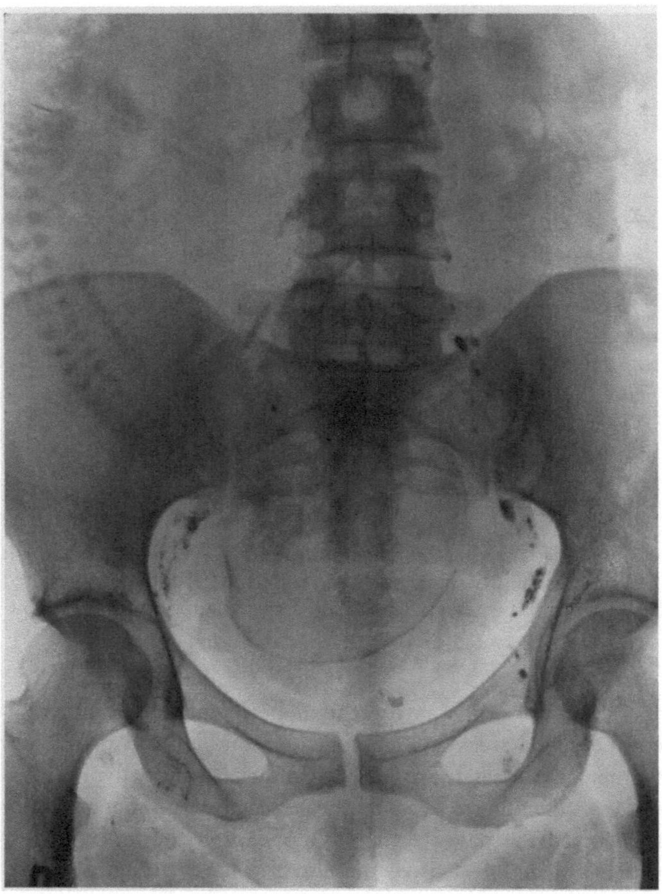

Fig. 6.11. Radiograph of the abdomen at the term of pregnancy, 2 years after E.R.T. in a woman with Hodgkin's disease. The patient had transitory amenorrhea for 8 months. With the return of the normal menstrual cycle, she was able to become pregnant and gave birth to a normal live foetus. Traces of Lipiodol are still present in the retroperitoneal lymph-nodes

amenorrhea proved to be transitory and regular menses returned after varying intervals of time. In this connection, we think it useful and interesting to note that five women with HD who had transistory amenorrhea were able, with the return of the normal menstrual cycle, to become pregnant and give birth to a normal live fetus at term (Fig. 6.11).

In some cases we saw a mild and transient lymphopenia but we never found a depression of bone-marrow function [10].

We have not observed any signs of intolerance to Lipiodol or to the dye [5, 22—24].

References

1. Bagliani, G., Chiappa, S., Galli, G.: Alcune considerazioni sulla pericolosità della linfadenografia diretta. Radiol. med. (Torino) **50**, 843 (1964).
2. Bousser, M. G.: Les accidents de la lymphographie. Sem. Hôp. (Paris) **68**, 1658 (1968).
3. Bron, K. M., Baum, S., Abrams, M. L.: Oil embolism in lymphangiography: incidence, manifestations and mechanism. Radiology **80**, 194 (1963).
4. Clouse, M. E., Mallgrimsson, J., Wenlund, D. E.: Complications following lymhography with particular reference to pulmonary oil embolism. Amer. J. Roentgenol. **96**, 972 (1966).
5. Collard, M., Collette, J. M.: Les modalités clinique de l'allergie au bleu patente violet. J. belge Radiol. **50**, 407 (1967).
6. Dargent, M., Chassard, I. L., Pommateau, E., Samin, F.: Echecs et complications de la lymphographie en cancérologie. Lyon chir. **58**, 309 (1962).
7. Davidson, J. W.: Lipid embolism to the brain following lymphography; case report and experimental study. Amer. J. Roentgenol. **105**, 763 (1969).
8. Desprez-Curely, J. P., Bismuth, V.: Accidents et incidents de la lymphographie. Ann. Radiol. **5**, 577 (1962).
9. Dolan, P. A.: Lymphography: complications encountered in 522 examinations. Radiology **86**, 876 (1966).
10. Edwards, J. M., Lloyd-Davies, J. E., Kinmonth, J. B.: Selective lymphogenia in man after intralymphatic injection of ^{131}I Lipiodol. Brit. med. J. **1967 I**, 331.
11. Fraimow, W., Wallance, S., Lewis, P., Greening, R. R., Cathchart, R. T.: Changes in pulmonary function due to lymphangiography. Radiology **85**, 231 (1965).
12. — — Greening, R. R., Cathchart, R. T.: Pulmonary function studies after lymphography. Cancer Chemother. Rep. **52**, 99 (1968).
13. Fucles, W. A.: Complications in lymphography with oily contrast media. Acta Radiol. **57**, 427 (1962).
14. Gilchrist, M. R.: Lymphangiography: a local evaluation. Minn. Med. **48**, 1000 (1965).
15. Gold, W. M., Youker, J., Anderson, S., Nadel, J. A.: Pulmonary-function abnormalities after lymphangiography. New Engl. J. Med. **273**, 519 (1965).
16. Goldberg, M. E., Feinberg, S. B.: Pulmonary infarction following lymphangiography in dogs: its implication in human studies. Radiology **81**, 479 (1963).
17. Gough, J. H., Gough, M. M., Thomas, M. L.: Pulmonary complications following lymphography. Brit. J. Radiol. **37**, 416 (1964).
18. Hallgrinsson, J., Clouse, M. E.: Pulmonary oil emboli after lymphangiography. Arch. Path. **80**, 426 (1965).
19. Ishida, O., Yoshihiro, T., Mori, S., Uchida, M.: Chest radiograms following lymphography with special reference to oil embolism. Med. J. Osaka Univ. **14**, 275 (1964).
20. Johansson, S., Sternby N. H., Theander, G., Wehlin, L.: Iodinated oil emulsion for lymphography. Acta Radiol. **4**, 690 (1965).
21. Koehler, P. R.: Lymphography. Complications and accidents. Proceedings of Lymphology. Ed.: A. Ruttiman. Stuttgart: G. Thieme 1966, p. 306.

22. Koehler, P. R.: Complications of lymphography. Lymphology 1, 116 (1968).
23. — Typical fatal reactions after lymphography. Cancer Chemother. Rep. 52, 113 (1968).
24. Kopp, W. L.: Anaphylaxis from Alphazurine 2 G during lymphography. J. Amer. med. Ass. 198, 668 (1966).
25. Kraus, R., Klemencic, J.: Vermeidbare Komplikationen bei Lymphographien. Med. Welt 15, 958 (1968).
26. Kunitsch, G., Holsten, D. R.: Erfahrungsbericht über 429 Lymphographien bei Geschwulstkranken. Med. Welt 4, 239 (1968).
27. Lewis, F. B., Schwartz, R., Dameshek, W.: X-radiations and alkylating agents as possible "trigger" mechanism in the autoimmune complications of malignant lymphoproliferative disease. Clin. exp. Immunol. 1, 3 (1966).
28. Nelson, B., Rush, E. A., Takasugy, M., Wittenberg, J.: Lipid embolism to the brain after lymphography. New Engl. J. med. 273, 1132 (1965).
29. Redman, H. C.: Dermatitis as a complication of lymphangiography. Radiology 86, 323 (1966).
30. Savoie, J. C., Gennes, J. L., Michard, J. R., Decourt, J.: Etude de deux cas de troubles acquis de l'hormogénèse thyroidienne à la suite d'injection d'huiles iodées. Ann. Endocr. 23, 293 (1962).
31. Secchi, G. C., Severini, A.: Modificazioni dell'attività funzionale del fegato dopo radioterapia endolinfatica con Lipiodol F ^{131}I. Radiol. med. (Torino) 51, 1277 (1965).
32. Takahashi, M., Abrams, H. L.: Arborizing pulmonary embolization following lymphangiography: report of three cases and experimental studies. Radiology 89, 633 (1967).
33. Threefoot, S. A.: Pulmonary hazards of lymphography. Cancer Chemother. Rep. 52, 107 (1968).
34. Weg, J. G., Harklevad, L. E.: Aberrations in pulmonary function due to lymphangiography. Dis. Chest. 53, 534 (1968).

Chapter 7

Results of Endolymphatic Radiotherapy: Histological Aspects

Federico Pizzetti and Umberto Veronesi

With 14 Figures

The histological aspects of lymph nodes after lymphography with radioactive Lipiodol are well known from a previous investigation made by Pizzetti et al. [5]. Such histological experience, however, relates to lymph nodes which either were not invaded by tumors or were infiltrated by metastases of carcinomas, especially from the bladder or uterus or malignant melanoma [1, 4, 6]. So far no extensive reports have been published on the direct action of radioactive Lipiodol on lymph nodes involving malignant lymphomas [2, 3]. With the aim of making a further contribution to this knowledge, we studied the retroperitoneal lymph nodes in patients with lymphoma who have undergone radioactive lymphography, and subsequently, a post mortem examination or a lymphadenectomy.

In order to establish the extent and the various aspects of the action of a radioactive isotope on lymph nodes involving malignant lymphoma, it is necessary to overcome an initial difficulty, i. e. to ascertain that the lymph node under examination had really been invaded by lymphoma cells. This is easy in cases where the radioactive Lipiodol has destroyed only a small part of the lymph node, leaving evident neoplastic residues, but our experience has shown that this occurrence is not very frequent. It is more difficult to make a diagnosis when there is extensive or total regression of the tumour as a result of irradiation (which seems to be the case in most instances) but it is obviously not feasible to provide diagnostic evidence of regression in the lymphomatous lesion.

It is not always easy to find a few cells that are definitely malignant in a lymph node that has been irradiated and is totally deranged in its histological structure. The diagnosis should then be based on other microscopic data, of which we will give details, based on our experience with the cases we have had under observation.

In general, when the X-ray film shows a clear-cut shrinkage of a lymph node with the passing of time, we may presume that the lymph node was originally invaded by the lymphoma and that the tumour has regressed as a result of the irradiation. This finding is of little significance if referred to a single lymph node or to just a few lymph nodes, but it would, naturally, be important if the shrinkage is related to numerous lymph nodes.

Nevertheless, a careful microscopic observation of the lymph nodes, even in the total absence of residual lesions, can also provide useful data in diagnosing regression of a lymphomatous alteration. A normal lymph node presents, as we have seen, typical histological findings after impregnation with radioactive Lipiodol. In lymph nodes of patients with lymphoma, the histological finding after radioactive lymphography is different, and presents certain characteristics that enable us to confirm the existence of a lymphomatous alteration that has regressed following irradiation.

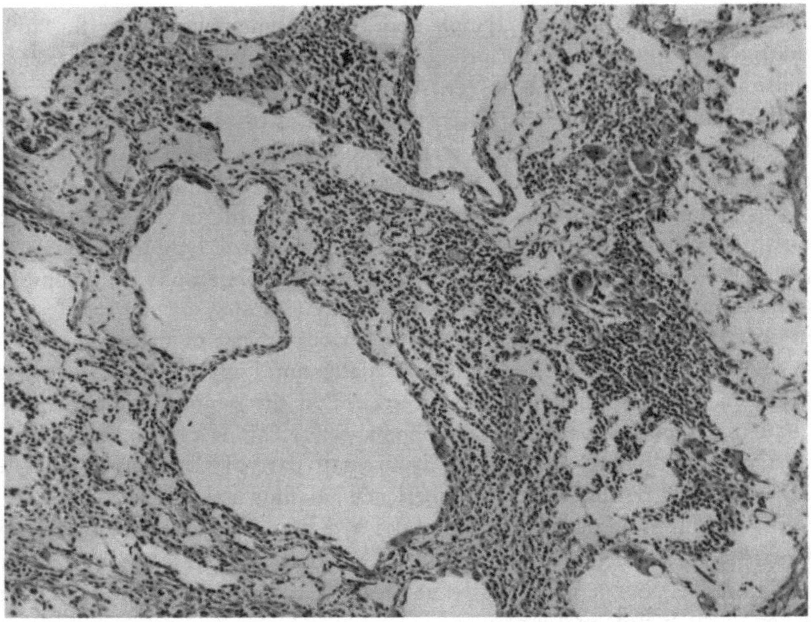

Fig. 7.1. Early alterations through radioactive Lipiodol in a normal lymph node. Material removed from a patient affected by carcinoma of the bladder during operation. Vacuoles caused by Lipiodol, initial lymphatic depletion

In this connection, it is useful to recall, by way of comparison, the type of lesions produced by ^{131}I on normal lymph nodes. Shortly after lymphography, a lymph node, slightly magnified under the microscope, has a "worm-eaten" appearance caused by small vacuoles that vary in diameter and number and are apparently separated by lymphatic tissue that is still rich in cells. The vacuoles are lined with round or flattened hystiocytes and with characteristic giant cells rich in nuclei (Fig. 7.1).

About two weeks after administration of Lipiodol ^{131}I the lymphatic tissue becomes less cellular and some fibroblasts appear in it, whilst the giant cells around the lumen of the vacuoles are more numerous and contain more nuclei. About one month later, the lymphatic tissue disappears almost completely and is replaced, between one vacuole and the other, by a sclerotic connective tissue containing a few fibroblasts (Fig. 7.2). After two months only thin shreds of sclero-hyaline connective tissue are left between the vacuoles. These alterations do not affect all lymph nodes of the same group or of nearby groups, nor even sometimes the whole lymph node, which may still contain areas of lymphatic tissue that is slightly damaged or even normal (Fig. 7.3). In general, our experience is that in normal lymph nodes, few areas are spared by the destructive and sclerosing action of Lipiodol; thus, the percentage of normal lymph nodes spared by the action of the isotope averages about 5%.

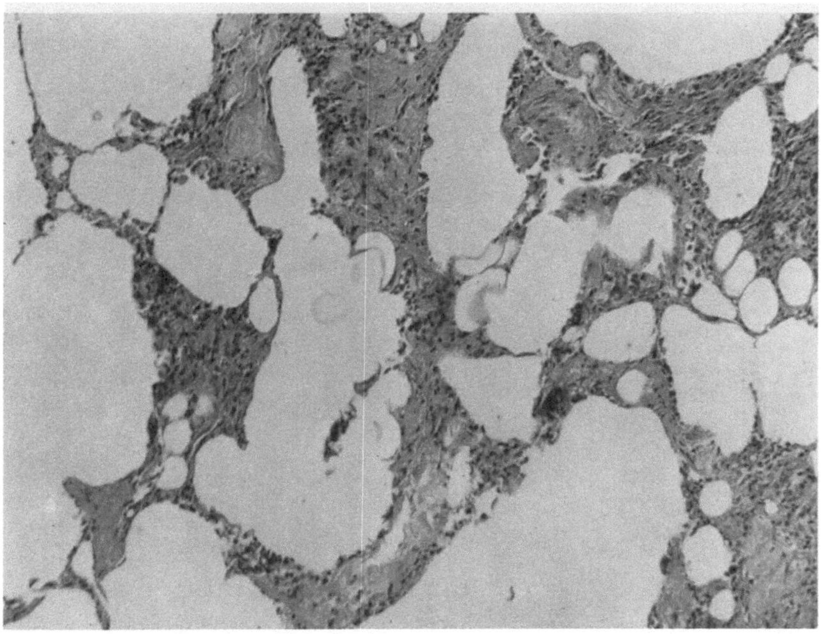

Fig. 7.2. Alterations due to Lipiodol in a normal lymph node one month after E.R.T. Material removed during operation from a patient affected by carcinoma of the bladder. Lymphatic tissue substituted by fibro-sclerotic connective with few fibroblasts; abundant vacuoles from Lipiodol

On comparing these histological findings with those observed in lymph nodes of patients with malignant lymphoma, in whom a marked shrinkage occurred following irradiation with Lipiodol ^{131}I, it can be observed that there are significant differences. First, the number and dimensions of the vacuoles caused by Lipiodol appear smaller than those seen in normal lymph nodes. Secondly, it is exceptional to find residues of normal lymphatic tissue between the vacuoles. This obviously means that there was no normal lymphatic tissue before irradiation with Lipiodol. Another feature worthy of note concerns the fibrous tissue, evolving towards sclerosis and hyalinosis, that remains among the vacuoles. This connective tissue always contains more fibroblasts than in normal lymph nodes; the fibroblast are sometimes found in short irregular bunches and are also associated with histiocytes (Figs. 7.4 and 7.5).

It should also be noted that some small areas of an amorphous hyaline substance (Fig. 7.6) and small hyaline blood vessels (Fig. 7.7) are present in these lymph nodes. In the preparations we have examined, which comprise material from both autopsies and operations, we frequently found lymph nodes presenting only the alterations described above, and in which the diagnosis of previous lymphomatous lesion is based on radiographic shrinkage in addition to evidence of these characteristic alterations in the phase following irradiation. In other lymph nodes, on the contrary, one may find residues of lymphomatous tissue, at times profoundly altered by the isotope. In these cases, naturally, evidence of a previous lymphomatous disease cannot be doubted.

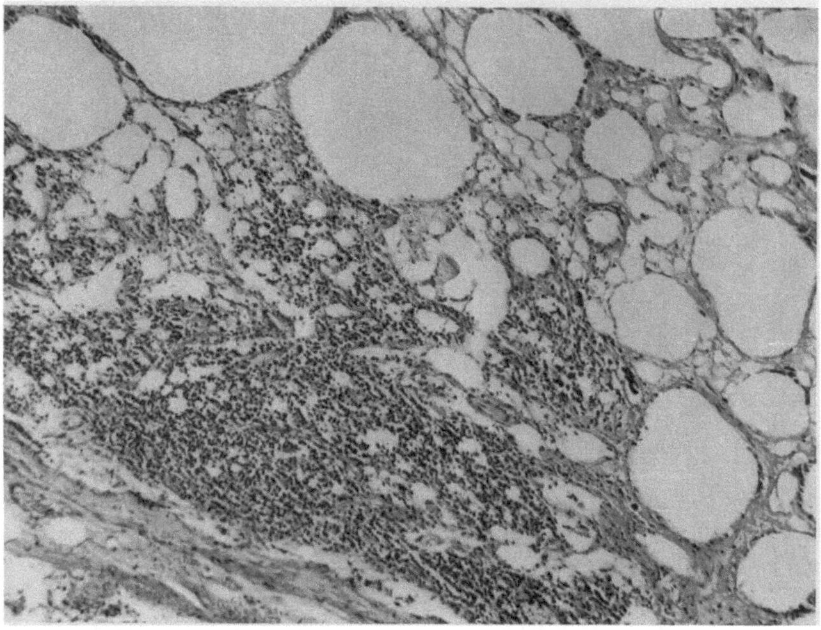

Fig. 7.3. Alterations due to Lipiodol in a normal lymph node. Material removed from patient affected by carcinoma of the bladder during operation. Residues of lymphatic tissue in an area not penetrated by radioactive Lipiodol

The presence of these tumour residues is perhaps more evident in lymphosarcoma, where one may note few clusters of atypical hyperchromic lymphatic cells (Figs. 7.7 and 7.8), than in reticulum cell sarcoma (Fig. 7.9) and in Hodgkin's disease. In the latter only a few large atypical cells can be observed, in which the characteristics of Sternberg's cell rarely remain unimpaired. Therefore we think that the destructive action of radioactive Lipiodol on lymphomatous lymph nodes may be said to be proven from a histologic, as well a radiographic point of view, even when the degree of destruction in a lymph node is such that it is not possible to evidence it with absolute certainty on the basis of microscopic reports only (Figs. 7.10, 7.11, 7.12).

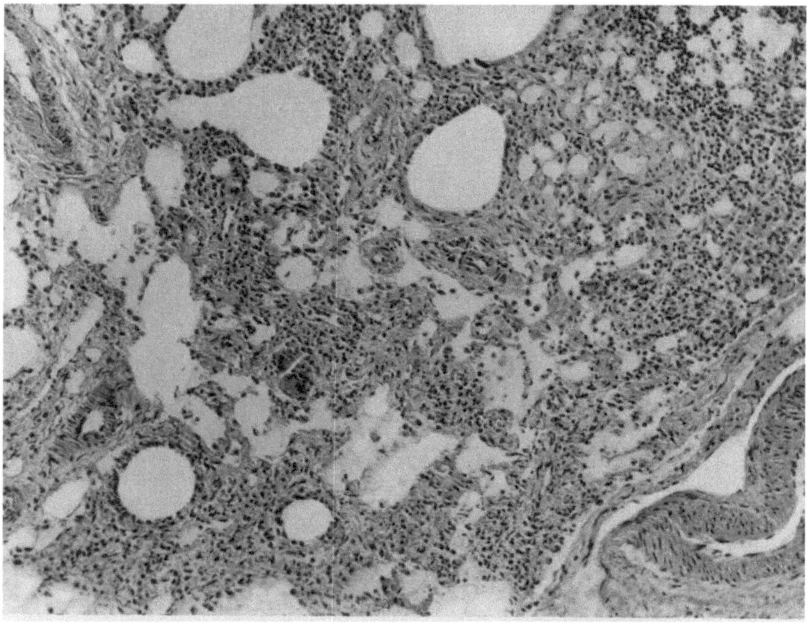

Fig. 7.4. Lymph node removed from patient affected by lymphosarcoma. Material removed during operation. Small and not very abundant vacuoles due to Lipiodol. Abundant tissue found between the vacuoles, rich in fibroblasts, with histiocytes and lymphatic cells of normal appearance

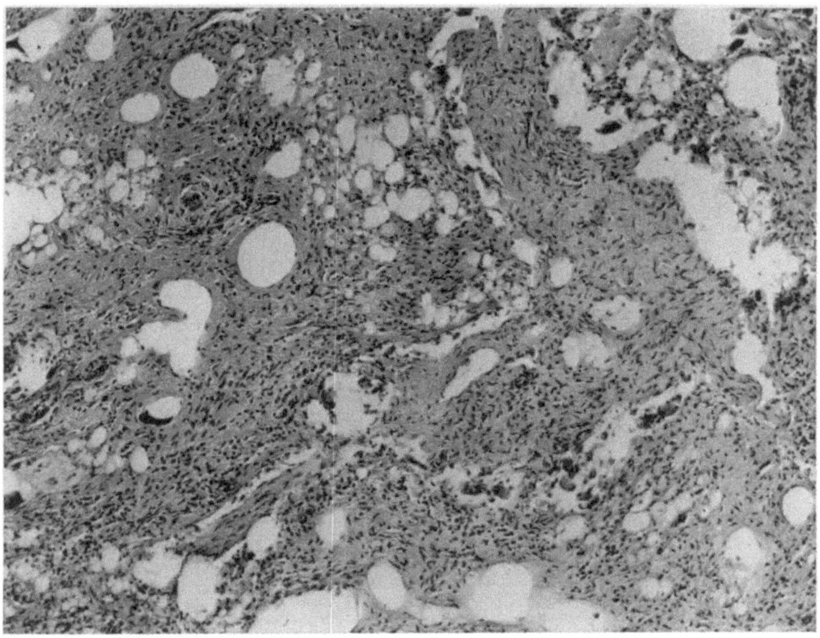

Fig. 7.5. Lymph node removed from patient affected by Hodgkin's disease. Material removed during operation. Abundant tissue found between the vacuoles, rich in fibroblasts

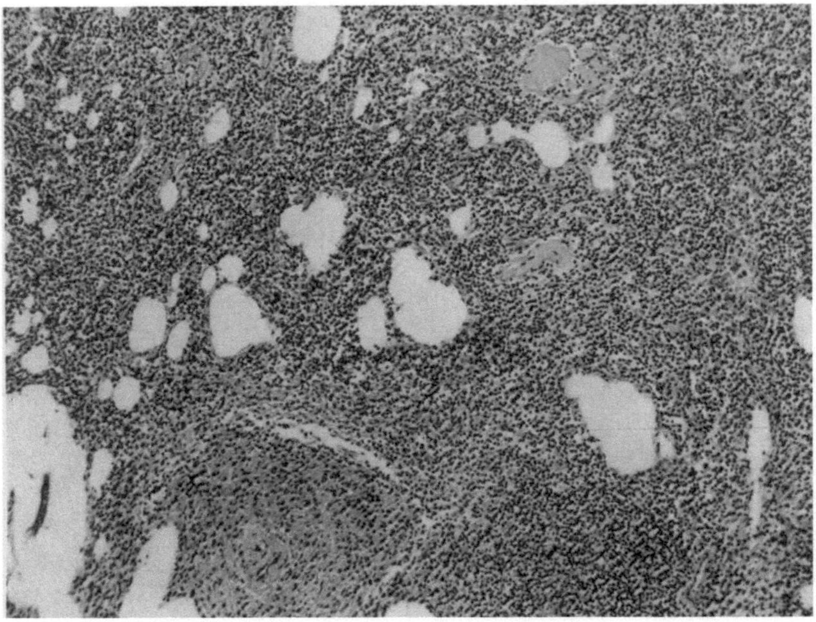

Fig. 7.6. Lymph node removed during operation from patient affected by lymphosarcoma. Thick lymphocellular infiltration without evident nuclear abnormalities. Presence of areas of amorphous hyaline substance

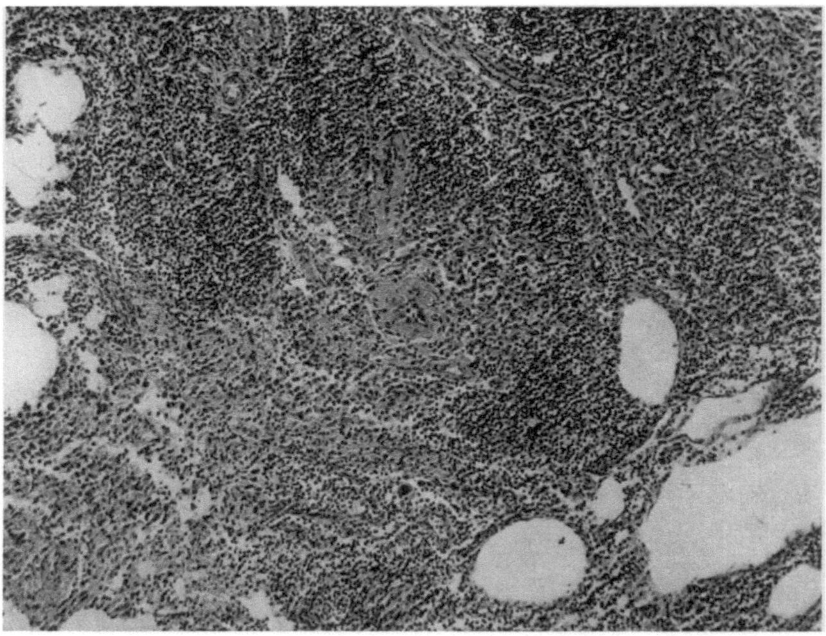

Fig. 7.7. Lymph node removed from patient affected by lymphosarcoma. Material removed during operation. Presence of small blood vessel with hyaline wall. Some nuclear abnormalities in the thick lymphocellular filtrate

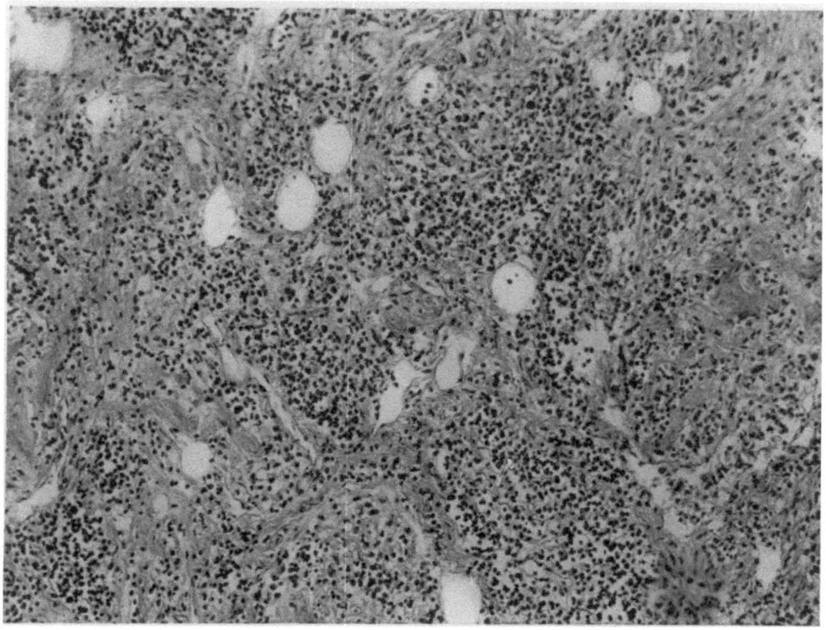

Fig. 7.8. Lymph node removed during operation from the same patient as shown in Fig. 7.6 and 7.7. The cells of the lymphosarcoma appear dissociated owing to proliferation of the fibrous connective tissue

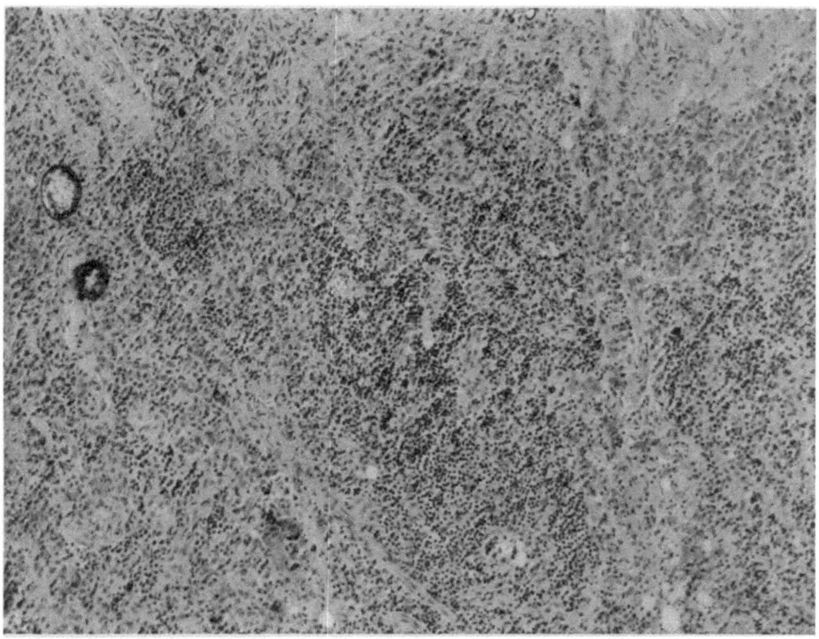

Fig. 7.9. Lymph node removed one year after administration of E.R.T. from patient affected by reticulum cell sarcoma. Autopsy material. Clusters of hyperchromic cells and extensive proliferation of histiocytes with no evident nuclear abnormalities

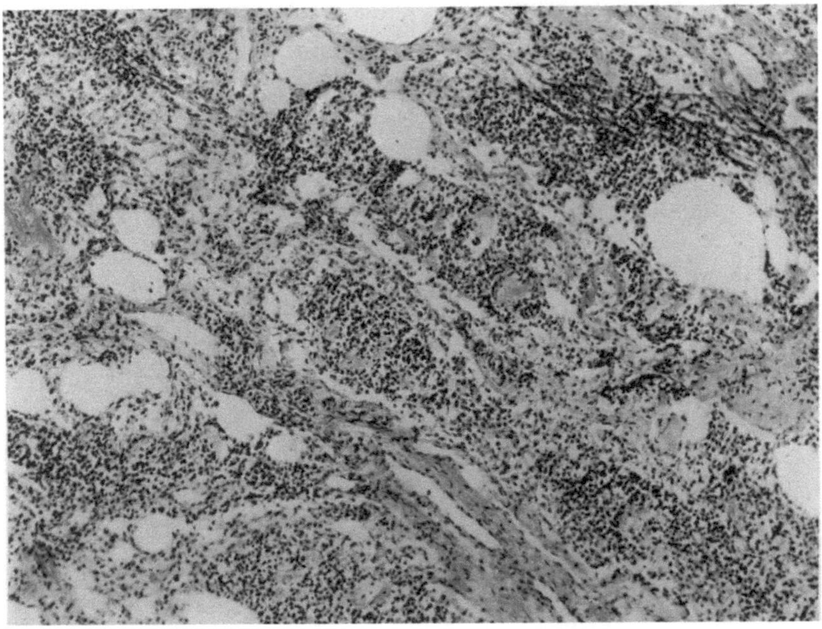

Fig. 7.10. Lymph node removed one year after E.R.T. from patient affected by lymphosarcoma. Autopsy material. Findings of uncertain interpretation: probable residues of lymphomatous tissue

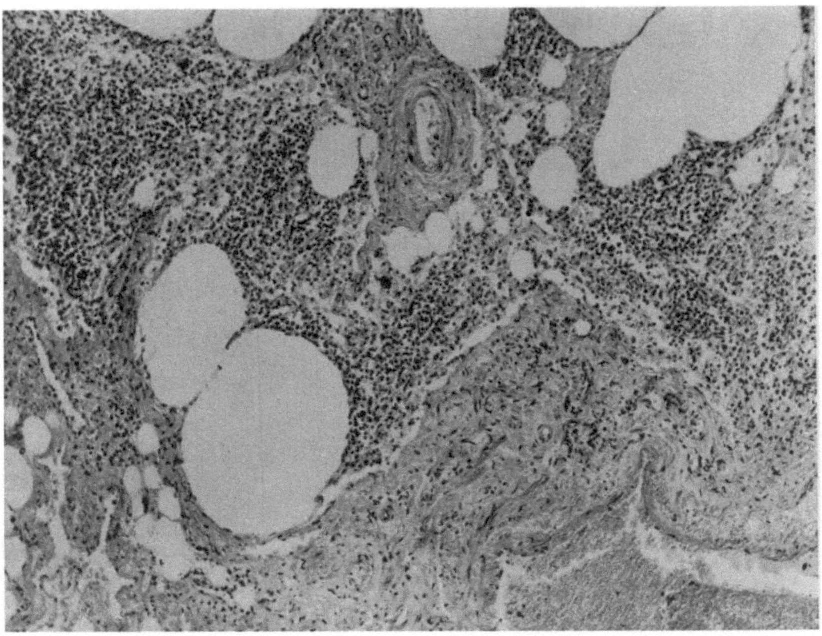

Fig. 7.11. Lymph node removed from patient affected by Hodgkin's disease, five months after E.R.T. Autopsy material. Histologically, the presence of lymphoma residues should be considered probable

The problem that concerns the pathologist is not only that of the morphological effects of irradiation; it is also necessary to ascertain the entity of such effects and their duration in time. With regard to the first of these two problems, the data we have to work on are limited, as they relate only to two cases of lymphadenectomy and four necropsy reports on patients in whom the destructive action of Lipiodol on the lymph nodes has been observed. On the basis of studies made on the two cases that were operated on, we can state that, at least temporarily, the extent of the destruction of the neoplastic tissue is remarkable. In the first of these two cases (lymphosarcoma) 14 lymph nodes were found with obvious residues—even if limited—of lymphomatous tissue, 2 with very little residue of the tumour, and 10 in which it could be presumed—on the basis of the histological data already referred to—that a lymphomatous lesion had existed (Fig. 7.12). In the second case (Hodgkin's disease) 6 lymph nodes were found with obvious residues of lymphoma cells (Fig. 7.13), 4 lymph nodes with little residues, 4 with the typical alterations caused by Lipiodol in normal lymph nodes (Fig. 7.14) and 13 with lesions that led us to presume complete destruction of a pre-existent malignant granuloma.

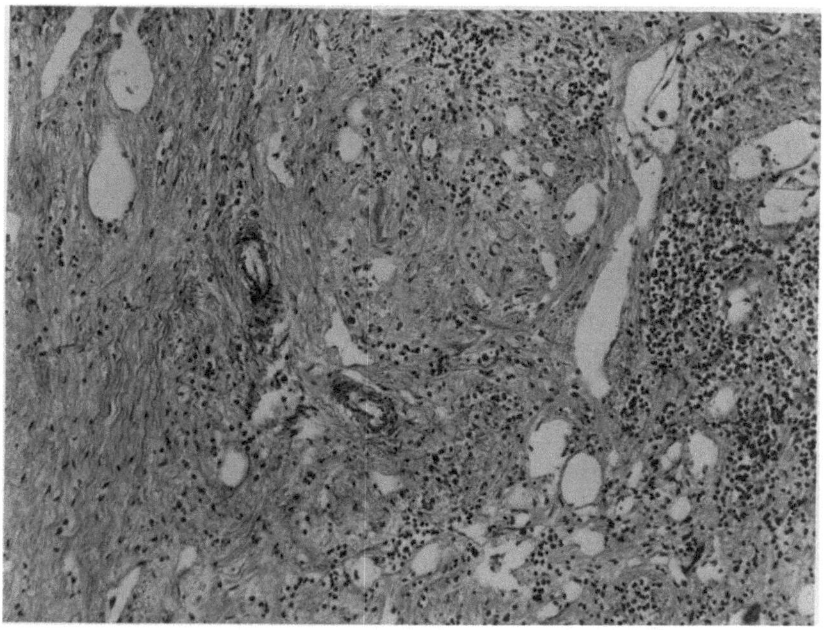

Fig. 7.12. Lymph node removed from patient affected by lymphosarcoma. Material removed during operation. Case difficult to interpret histologically: sparse residues of lymphoma?

Even considering these last features in which there is no certain proof of the destructive action of radioactive Lipiodol in a critical spirit, the results of an examination of the two operated patients are such that we feel justified in stating that radioactive lymphography has a positive therapeutic action on malignant

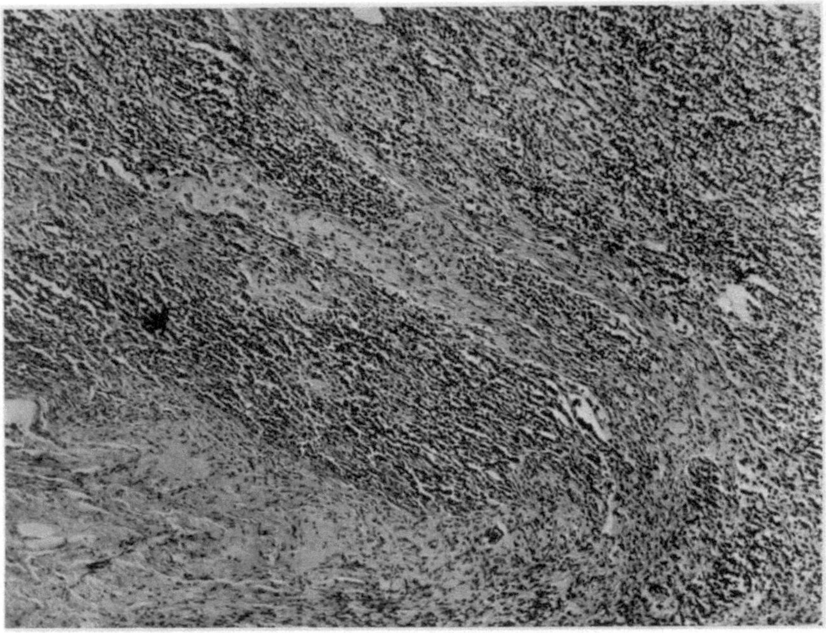

Fig. 7.13. Lymph node removed from patient affected by Hodgkin's disease. Material removed during operation. Lymphoma in active phase

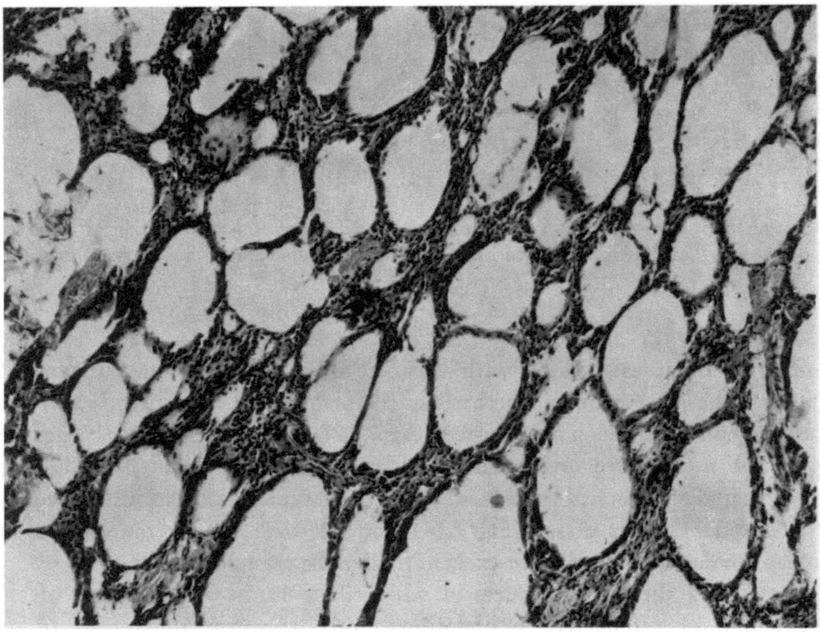

Fig. 7.14. Lymph node removed from patient affected by Hodgkin's disease. Alterations due to Lipiodol, similar to those found in normal lymph nodes

lymphomas. In these cases one can observe—as a result of irradiation—destruction of the lymphomatous tissue to a greater or lesser extent, its substitution by fibroblasts and histiocytes, and a tendency to sclerosis and hyalinosis, which can create conditions preventing the survival of residues of lymphoma.

With regard to the second problem, the duration of the therapeutic action of Lipiodol ^{131}I, this may be dealt with on the basis of data from the autopsy findings in eight patients who died as a result of malignant lymphoma, in a period of 5 months to one year after E.R.T. (3 cases of Hd, 3 cases of LSA, 2 cases of RSA). In four of these cases we found lymph nodes with alterations indicating the regression of a lymphoma, alongside lymph nodes affected by a lymphoma still in an active phase. In four other cases, however, the lymphoma tissue seemed free of alterations in all the lymph nodes that were examined, in which no vacuoles caused by Lipiodol were found.

In this instance, it becomes necessary to discuss the meaning of this last finding, for which there are two explanations: a recurrence of the malignant lymphoma some time after treatment, or the fact that the radioactive Lipiodol has failed to penetrate into the lymph node. Some lymph nodes with scanty alterations due to Lipiodol were found in the surgical material, while alterations due to Lipiodol have been found on autopsy in the case of a patient who underwent lymphography one year before decease; thus, we can consider that there is some foundation for the hypothesis that the persistence of the tumour depends mainly, if not exclusively, on the failure of the isotope to penetrate the pathological lymph node or to penetrate it completely. This interpretation is also supported by evidence [5] that, in cases of lymph node metastases of epithelial tumours, destructive action takes place only in the smaller metastases, that do not prevent penetration by the isotope, whilst it is ineffective in lymph nodes that are totally invaded by the neoplastic tissue.

Finally, on the basis of our case material, which is numerically limited but morphologically enlightening, we can state that destructive action by radioactive Lipiodol on malignant lymphomas certainly exists and that it can reach a remarkable extent in cases where the Lipiodol has readily penetrated the lymph node. In this cases, the lymphomatous tissue is destroyed and substituted by a proliferation of fibroblasts with a subsequent evolution toward sclerosis and hyalinosis. This causes a marked reduction in the volume of the lymph nodes, that can clearly be seen radiographically some time after lymphography. The effect, however, is not achieved in lymph nodes into which the Lipiodol has not penetrated, owing to occlusion of the afferent lymphatic vessels due to a complete lymphomatous transformation of the lymph node.

This finding justifies the systematic use of radioactive lymphography in patients affected by malignant lymphoma in the initial stages. If performed in the early stages of the disease, as was done in the two cases that were operated on for a check-up, lymphography, in fact, with easy penetration of Lipiodol into many lymph nodes, causes destruction of the lymphoma cells to a greater or lesser extent. In the material removed by us during operations, none of the lymph nodes we examined were entirely free of vacuoles caused by Lipiodol, and it was found that penetration of the isotope was marginal (hence with little therapeutic effect) in only two lymph nodes in the case of LSA and six in the case of Hd.

With regard to the side effects of irradiation with E.R.T., we can report that we found no fibrosis of the hepatic and pulmonary tissues in any of the 8 cases where a complete post mortem investigation was possible [2].

References

1. Ariel, I. M.: Lymphography and endolymphatic administration of radioactive isotopes for treating cancer. N. Y. St. J. Med. **68**, 1247 (1968).
2. Bonadonna, G., Chiappa, S., Musumeci, R., Uslenghi, C.: Endolymphatic radiotherapy in malignant lymphomas. A clinical evaluation of 285 patients. Cancer **22**, 885 (1968).
3. Chiappa, S., Galli, G., Guarino, M., Barbaini, S., Ravasi, G.: Prime osservazioni istologiche di linforeticolopatie sistemiche trattate con Lipiodol ^{131}I per via endolinfatica. Tumori **49**, 87 (1963).
4. — — Luciani, L., Severini, A., Talamazzi, F.: La radioterapia endolinfatica nel trattamento delle metastasi da carcinoma dell'utero. Minerva Ginec. **16**, 487 (1964).
5. Mattea, E., Chiappa, S., Pizzetti, F., Bono, A. V., Galli, G.: La radioterapia endolinfatica con Lipiodol F ^{131}I nel carcinoma della vescica. Urologia **31**, 167 (1964).
6. — Bono, A. V., Chiappa, S., Galli, G., Severini, A., Arrigoni, G.: Linfoadenografia e radioterapia endolinfatica nelle metastasi da neoplasie della sfera urologica. Relaz. Uff. XXXVII Congr. Soc. It. Urol. Ed. Novograf. Milano 1964.

Chapter 8

Endolymphatic Radiotherapy in Relation to other Treatments for Malignant Lymphomas

S. CHIAPPA, R. MUSUMECI, and C. USLENGHI

With 2 Figures

The salient features of E.R.T. with Lipiodol ^{131}I have been described by CHIAPPA et al. in numerous publications [6, 8]. They may be summarized as follows:

1. it is single-session treatment that can, if necessary, be repeated after a short interval;

2. high tissue doses can be given without harmful side-effects in the majority of cases;

3. with exclusion of a mild and transient lymphopenia, the treatment does not depress bone-marrow function [10];

4. E.R.T. does not exclude a complementary course of external therapy, usually T.C.T., to inadequately filled lymph nodes.

At this juncture it is worth outlining the main points of difference between the routine therapies for malignant lymphomas, namely transcutaneous radiotherapy and chemotherapy on the one hand, and E.R.T. on the other [1, 5, 7, 8].

Endolymphatic injection of the radioactive contrast medium (E.R.T.) offers the following advantages over transcutaneous radiotherapy [8]:

1. the lymph nodes are irradiated from the inside at very high doses;

2. irradiation of confined to the lymph node, partly because the radiation source is located inside it and partly because the nuclide we use is such that the dose absorbed is mainly in the form of beta radiations, which are known to have a short passage through the tissues. Hence irradiation of neighboring tissues is negligible and the volume/dose minimal. This is a great advantage when treating pelvic lymph nodes that are contiguous with highly radiosensitive organs, such as the ovaries;

3. several lymph node groups spread over a large area are irradiated simultaneously. This advantage is the more appreciable when we consider that transcutaneous radiotherapy can cause trouble when the pelvic and retroperitoneal lymph nodes have to be treated;

a

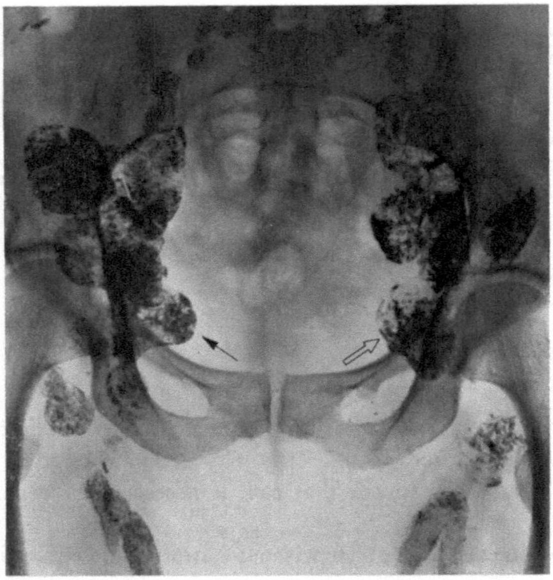

Fig. 8.1. Patient with lymphosarcoma. a Film taken 24 h after lymphography (10 ml of Lipiodol F on the right side and 10 ml of Lipiodol ^{131}I on the left side). All the lymph nodes (white and black arrows) are involved

b

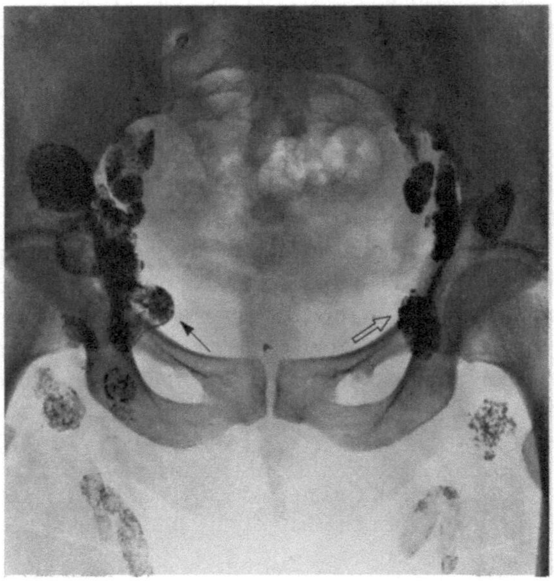

b Follow-up film 47 days after lymphography: during this time a course of chemotherapy (HN_2) was administered. Shrinkage of the lymph nodes on the left side (white arrow-^{131}I) is evident. Even involved lymph nodes on the right side (black arrow-HN2) are smaller

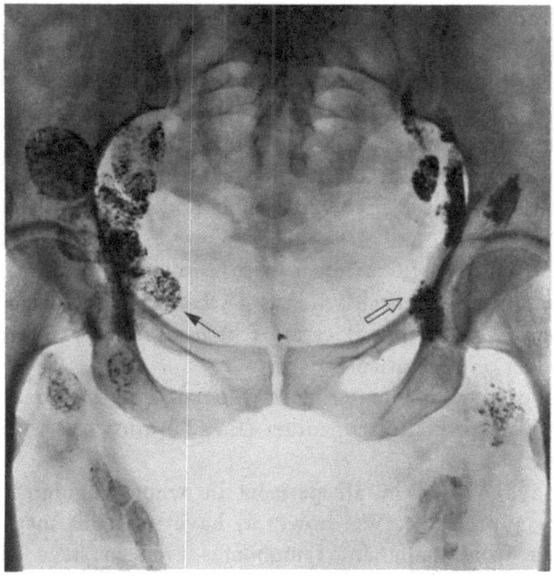

c

c Follow-up film 167 days after lymphography: good shrinkage on the left side (white arrow-^{131}I). Progression of the disease on the right side (black arrow-HN2)

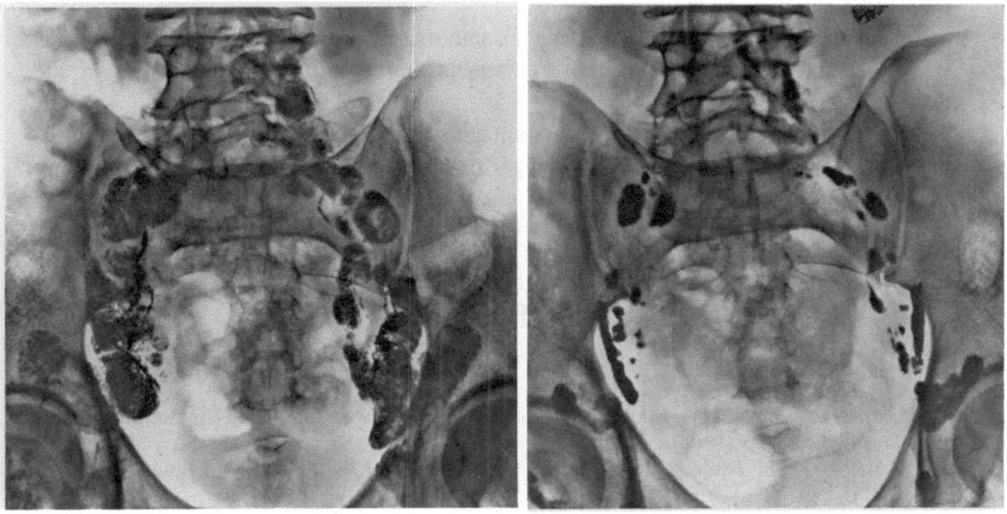

a b

Fig. 8.2. Patient with Hodgkin's disease. a Film taken 24 h after lymphography (10 ml of Lipiodol ^{131}I on the right side and 10 ml of Lipiodol F on the left side). All the lymph nodes are involved. b Follow-up film 60 days after lymphography. On the left side external TCT was administered (3500 rad within 4 weeks). Good shrinkage of all pathological lymph nodes in both sides

4. one final advantage is that the complete therapy can be given in a single session and the case can be followed up as an outpatients.

E.R.T. has the following advantages over systemic chemotheray [2—4, 9, 11—16]:

1. it has a minimal effect on the blood pattern: the patients we treated and followed up systematically with repeated cell counts and Hb tests at no time showed any appreciable change attributable to the treatment, even in the leukocytes;

2. the local effect on the involved lymph nodes seems to be more intense and more lasting;

3. a complete course of treatment with chemotherapeutic agents can only be repeated after a suitable interval, whereas a second injection of radioactive contrast medium has been given in special cases as little as 10 days after the first, without any untoward effect on the patient.

The analysis of our case material of 426 patients with malignant lymphomas treated with radioactive contrast medium (E.R.T.) allows us to make the following general statements:

1. E.R.T. may be used in all patients in whom inguino-iliac or para-aortic adenopathies are appreciable. We, however, have used this method in virtually all patients suffering from malignant lymphomas even in stage I_1 because we have found that retroperitoneal lymph nodes can often be involved without giving clinical evidence.

2. The local effect. viz. the shrinkage of the lymph nodes, takes place after variable intervals accordings to the disease. For HD, shrinkage usually begins 1—2 weeks after injection of the radioactive contrast medium and reaches its maximum within 2—4 months. In LSA and RSA, shrinkage starts sooner, even within a week, and reaches its maximum within 20 days.

3. The therapeutic effect of the radioactive contrast medium is proportional to the degree of filling of the lymph nodes.

4. The local results are associated in some cases with remission of the general symptoms, the remission being more or less lasting according to the spread of the disease.

As to a general comparative assessment, the effects of E.R.T. in the retroperitoneal lymph nodes are always superior to those obtained with chemotherapy [1, 5, 7] and, when the lymph nodes are well filled, apparently equal—on solely radiologic criteria—to those obtained with T.C.T. [8] (Figs. 8.1 and 8.2).

References

1. ARIEL, I. M., RESNICK, M. I., GALEY, D.: The intralymphatic administration of radioactive isotopes and cancer chemotherapeutic drugs. Surgery **55**, 355 (1964).
2. BATTEZZATI, M., TAGLIAFERRO, A., DONINI, I.: La via endolinfatica in terapia clinica. Gazz. Sanit. **33**, 3 (1962).
3. — — — Primi risultati della terapia endolinfatica. Riv. Emoter. Immunoemat. **9**, 23 (1962).
4. — DONINI, I.: Il sistema linfatico nella pratica clinica. Ed.: PICCIN. Padova 1968.
5. BONADONNA, G., CHIAPPA, S., DI PIETRO, S., MARANO, P., MOLINARI, R., USLENGHI, C.: L'association de la radiothérapie endolymphatique et des agents alkylants dans le traitement des hématosarcomes rétropéritonéaux. Nouv. Rev. franç. Hémat. **7**, 381 (1967).
6. CHIAPPA, S.: Il valore diagnostico e terapeutico dell'adenolinfografia. Atti Accad. Med. Lombarda **17**, 6 (1962).

7. Chiappa, S., Galli, G., Palmia, C.: Observations on intralymphatic radiotherapy and general chemotherapy. Clin. Radiol. **15**, 202 (1964).
8. — Bonadonna, G., Musumeci, R., Uslenghi, C.: Endolymphatic radiotherapy in malignant lymphomas. Long-term results. Lymphology **3**, 13 (1970).
9. Crispen, J. F., Jeffries, P. F.: Lymphangiography. A simple method of dye infusion. J. Amer. med. Ass. **182**, 872 (1962).
10. Edwards, J. M., Lloyd-Davies, J. E., Kinmonth, J. B.: Selective lymphopenia in man after intralymphatic injection of ^{131}I Lipiodol. Brit. med. J. **1967 I**, 331.
11. Goffrini, P., Rastelli, G. C.: L'introduzione di farmaci per via linfatica. Arch. ital. Chir. **87**, 181 (1961).
12. Jackson, L. G., Wallance, S., Weiss, A. J.: Chemiotherapy by intralymphatic infusion. Cancer **15**, 955 (1962).
13. Karnofsky, D. A.: Summary of results obtained with nitrogen mustard in the treatment of neoplastic disease. Ann. N.Y. Acad. Sci. **68**, 899 (1958).
14. — Burchenal, J. H., Ormsbee, R. A., Cornman, I., Rhoads, C. P.: Experimental observations on use of nitrogen mustards in treatment of neoplastic disease. Approaches to Tumor Chemotherapy AAAS: 293 (1947).
15. — Miller, D. G., Phillips, R. F.: Role of chemotherapy in the management of early Hodgkin's disease. Amer. J. Roentgenol. **90**, 968 (1963).
16. Pescetto, G.: Prospettive della chemioterapia intralinfatica nelle metastasi linfonodali del cancro uterino. Clin. Ostet. Ginec. **63**, 493 (1961).

Chapter 9

Conclusions

S. Chiappa, R. Musumeci, and C. Uslenghi

The experience achieved in our Institutes over about 8 years, treating by E.R.T. 426 cases of histologically proven malignant lymphomas, allows us to draw some critical conclusions.

It should nonetheless be made clear that, because of a series of circumstances connected partly with the manual procedures involved and partly with the distribution of the radioactive contrast medium in the lymph nodes, E.R.T. cannot be considered consistently radical. In fact, in about one-third of the patients to whom E.R.T. was given it was not possible to ensure uniform and adequate filling of the retroperitoneal node chains. For this reason it was necessary to resort to external T.C.T. in some cases. Further E.R.T. does not seem to comply with modern standards of radicality, especially at the level of the para-aortic chains, because the lymph nodes above the second lumbar vertebra usually fill poorly.

The total number of recurrences or new localizations of malignant lymphoma in the retroperitoneal node chains was fairly low in our series (about 12.2%). This number is, however, only approximate and is probably on the low side. Indeed, it is impossible to make a precise clinical assessment of the condition of the retroperitoneal node chains in all patients.

A highly positive feature is that only in a very few cases did new localizations of lymphomatous disease occur in lymph nodes that had initially been negative (Stages I and II). This shows that the dose of radiation administered to the lymph nodes was sufficient to destroy the microscopic foci of lymphomatous cells present and that probably all the lymph nodes were filled with Lipiodol ^{131}I.

For these reasons, in the light of current thinking on the irradiation of malignant lymphomas, which includes treatment fields over all the lymph node regions both above and below the diaphragm (mantle and inverted Y fields), and on the basis of our own and other investigators' experience, we consider that E.R.T. assumes a well-defined place.

In patients classified after lymphography in the first stages of the disease (I_1, I_2, II) and therefore with retroperitoneal node chains almost certainly not invaded by the malignant lymphoma, when the lymph nodes appear adequately filled by the Lipiodol ^{131}I, we use E.R.T. as we would use radiotherapy below the diaphragm. In these patients the radiotherapeutic treatment is completed with T.C.T. (mantle field) above the diaphragm. In such cases we consider E.R.T. to be as effective as the prophylactic extension of the treatment with external T.C.T. (inverted Y field).

In patients with primary onset of the disease below the diaphragm we administer E.R.T. for diagnostic purposes and then complete the treatment with external T.C.T.

In patients classified after lymphography in the third stage (III), in the majority of whom retroperitoneal node chains are invaded by lymphoma, and in patients in the first stages (I_1, I_2, II) in whom filling of the lymph nodes is not sufficiently homogeneous, we complete the treatment below the diaphragm with the classic inverted Y field extended to cover the spleen.

When treating patients classified after lymphography in the third stage (III) another problem can be resolved by using E.R.T. Since it is practically impossible to irradiate at the same time both upper and lower trunk mantles, the predominant site of the disease should be the deciding factor. Ordinarily, treatment to this region is carried to completion before irradiation is started to other lymphoid regions. This type of radiotherapeutic treatment is usually called "sequential technique" (see Chapter 1). In these cases we usually carry out the irradiation of the upper trunk lymphatics first, since the retroperitoneal adenopathies are opacified and irradiated with Lipiodol ^{131}I. After completion of the upper mantle, external T.C.T. is given to all lymphatic chains below the diaphragm. We think this a very useful characteristic of E.R.T.

Another very important, though purely palliative, use for E.R.T. is in stage IV patients with large retroperitoneal adenopathies, marked systemic signs and evidence of visceral compression. In these cases internal irradiation with Lipiodol ^{131}I (E.R.T.), as an adjunct to one or more courses of chemotherapy, ensures rapid shrinkage of the adenopathies and almost always gives remission of the systemic signs.

Subject Index

Monographs already Published

1 Schindler, R., Lausanne: Die tierische Zelle in Zellkultur. DM 16,—
2 Neuroblastomas — Biochemical Studies. Edited by C. Bohuon, Villejuif (Symposium). DM 16,—
3 Hueper, W. C., Bethesda: Occupational and Environmental Cancers of the Respiratory System. DM 34,—
4 Goldman, L., Cincinnati: Laser Cancer Research. DM 16,—
5 Metcalf, D., Melbourne: The Thymus. Its Role in Immune Responses, Leukaemia Development and Carcinogenesis. DM 24,—
6 Malignant Transformation by Viruses. Edited by W. H. Kirsten, Chicago (Symposium). DM 32,—
7 Moertel, Ch. G., Rochester: Multiple Primary Malignant Neoplasms. Their Incidence and Significance. DM 18,—
8 New Trends in the Treatment of Cancer. Edited by L. Manuila, S. Moles, and P. Rentchnick, Geneva. DM 32,—
9 Lindenmann, J., Zürich, and P. A. Klein, Gainesville/Florida: Immunological Aspects of Viral Oncolysis. DM 18,—
10 Nelson, R. S., Houston: Radioactive Phosphorus in the Diagnosis of Gastrointestinal Cancer. DM 15,—
11 Freeman, R. G., and J. M. Knox, Houston: Treatment of Skin Cancer. DM 15,—
12 Lynch, H. T., Houston: Hereditary Factors in Carcinoma. DM 24,—
13 Tumours in Children. Edited by H. B. Marsden, and J. K. Steward, Manchester. DM 72,—
14 Odartchenko, N., Lausanne: Production cellulaire érythropoïétique. DM 28,—
15 Sokoloff, B., Lakeland/Florida: Carcinoid and Serotonin. DM 24,—
16 Jacobs, M. L., Duarte/California: Malignant Lymphomas and their Management. DM 18,—
17 Normal and Malignant Cell Growth. Edited by R. J. M. Fry, Argonne, M. L. Griem, Argonne, and W. H. Kirsten, Chicago (Symposium). DM 56,80
18 Anglesio, E., Torino: The Treatment of Hodgkin's Disease. DM 24,—
19 Bannasch, P., Würzburg: The Cytoplasm of Hepatocytes during Carcinogenesis. DM 32,—
20 Rubidomycin. A new Agent against Leukemia. Edited by J. Bernard, R. Paul, M. Boiron, C. Jacquillat, and R. Maral, Paris. DM 48,—
21 Scientific Basis of Cancer Chemotherapy. Edited by G. Mathé, Villejuif (Symposium). DM 28,—
22 Koldovský, P., Philadelphia: Tumor Specific Transplantation Antigen. DM 24,—
23 Fuchs, W. A., Bern, J. W. Davidson, Toronto, and H. W. Fischer, Ann Arbor: Lymphography in Cancer. DM 76,—
24 Hayward, J. L., London: Hormonal Research in Human Breast Cancer. DM 34,—
25 Roy-Burman, P., Los Angeles: Analogues of Nucleic Acid Components. Mechanisms of Action. DM 28,—
26 Tumors of the Liver. Edited by G. T. Pack and A. H. Islami, New York. DM 56,—

27 Szymendera, J., Warsaw: Bone Mineral Metabolism in Cancer. DM 32,—

28 Meek, E. S., Bristol: Antitumour and Antiviral Substances of Natural Origin. DM 16,—

29 Aseptic Environments and Cancer Treatment. Edited by G. Mathé, Villejuif (Symposium). DM 22,—

30 Advances in the Treatment of Acute (Blastic) Leukemias. Edited by G. Mathé, Villejuif (Symposium). DM 38,—

31 Denoix, P., Villejuif: Treatment of Malignant Breast Tumors: Indications and Results. DM 48,—

32 Nelson, R. S., Houston: Endoscopy in Gastric Cancer. DM 48,—

33 Experimental and Clinical Effects of L-Asparaginase. Edited by E. Grundmann, Wuppertal-Elberfeld, and H. F. Oettgen, New York (Symposium). DM 58,—

34 Endo, H., Fukuoka, T. Ono, Tokyo, T. Sugimura, Tokyo: Chemistry and Biological Actions of 4-Nitroquinoline 1-oxide. DM 36,—

35 Penn, I., Denver: Malignant Tumors in Organ Transplant Recipients. DM 24,—

36 Current Concepts in the Management of Leukemia and Lymphoma. Edited by J. E. Ultmann, M. L. Griem, W. H. Kirsten, and R. W. Wissler, Chicago (Symposium) DM 48,—

37 Chiappa, S., R. Musumeci, and C. Uslenghi, Milano: Endolymphatic Radiotherapy in Malignant Lymphomas. DM 48,—

Special Supplement: Biology of Amphibian Tumors. Edited by M. Mizell, New Orleans. DM 86,—

In Preparation

Ackermann, N. B., Boston: Use of Radioisotopic Agents in the Diagnosis of Cancer

Boiron, M., Paris: The Viruses of the Leukemia-Sarcoma Complex

Cavaliere, R., A. Rossi-Fanelli, B. Mondovi, and G. Moricca, Roma: Selective Heat Sensitivity of Cancer Cells

Grundmann, E., Wuppertal-Elberfeld: Morphologie und Cytochemie der Carcinogenese

Irlin, I. S., Moskva: Mechanisms of Viral Carcinogenesis

Koller, P. C., London: The Role of Chromosomes in Cancer Biology

Langley, F. A., and A. C. Crompton, Manchester: Epithelial Abnormalities of the Cervix Uteri

Mathé, G., Villejuif: L'Immunothérapie des Cancers

Merkow, L., and M. Slifkin, Pittsburgh: Oncogenic Simian Adenoviruses

Parker, J., and R. J. Lukes, Los Angeles: Lymphocyte Transformation in Neoplastic Disease

Weil, R., Lausanne: Biological and Structural Properties of Polyoma Virus and its DNA

Williams, D. C., Oxted, Surrey: The Basis for Therapy of Hormon Sensitive Tumours

MIX
Papier aus verantwortungsvollen Quellen
Paper from responsible sources
FSC® C105338

If you have any concerns about our products,
you can contact us on
ProductSafety@springernature.com

In case Publisher is established outside the EU,
the EU authorized representative is:
Springer Nature Customer Service Center GmbH
Europaplatz 3, 69115 Heidelberg, Germany

Printed by Libri Plureos GmbH
in Hamburg, Germany